KETTLEBELL
SIMPLE & SINISTER

BY PAVEL

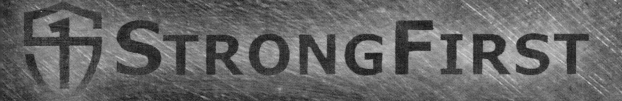

Published by StrongFirst, Inc.

9190 Double Diamond Parkway

Reno, NV 89521, USA

www.StrongFirst.com

Editor: Laree Draper • www.ontargetpublications.net

Photography: Ralph DeHaan Photography • www.ralphdehaan.com

and Teal Tree Studios, Inc. • www.tealtreestudios.com

Design: Rachel Darvas • rachel.darvas.sfg@gmail.com

Library of Congress Cataloging-in-Publication Data

Tsatsouline, Pavel

ISBN 978-0-9898924-0-7

I. Strength training. 2. Fitness. 3. Physical education and training.

DISCLAIMER

The author and publisher of this book are not responsible in any manner whatsoever for any injury that may occur through following the instructions contained in this material. The activities may be too strenuous or dangerous for some people. The readers should always consult a physician before engaging in them.

The author would like to thank the following ladies and gentlemen for their suggestions:

Michael Castrogiovanni, Andrea Chang, Ron Farrington, Steve Freides, Eric Frohardt, Dr. Kristann Heinz, Dan John, Rob Lawrence, Jeremy Layport, Geoff Neupert, Mark Reifkind, George Samuelson, Alexandre Senart, Mark Toomey, Chad Waterbury, David Whitley, Fabio Zonin, as well as a dozen gentlemen who chose to remain anonymous. A special thanks to Brandon Hetzler and Nikki Shlosser.

PART I: SIMPLE

PART II: SINISTER

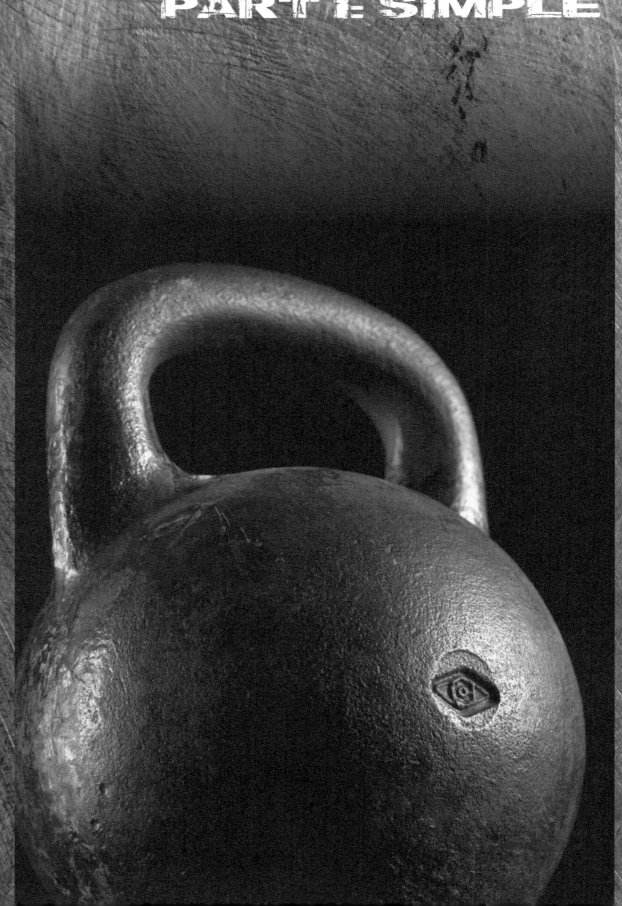

PART 1: SIMPLE

THE RUSSIAN KETTLEBELL --
AN EXTREME HANDHELD GYM

*If a kettlebell were a person, it would be the type of a guy
you would want [on your side] in an alley fight.*

—Glenn Buechlein, powerlifter

The kettlebell is an ancient Russian weapon against weakness.

Called *girya* in Russian, this cannonball with a handle has been making better men and women for over 300 years. In imperial Russia, "kettlebell" was synonymous with "strength." A strongman or weightlifter was called a *girevik* or a "kettlebell man." Strong ladies were *girevichkas* or "kettlebell women." "Not a single sport develops our muscular strength and bodies as well as kettlebell athletics," reported Russian magazine *Hercules* in 1913.

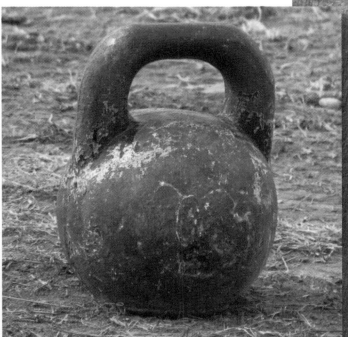

A kettlebell at the Vaziani Air Base Gym in the former Soviet republic of Georgia.

Photo courtesy of Lt. Col. Minter B. Ralston IV, USMC

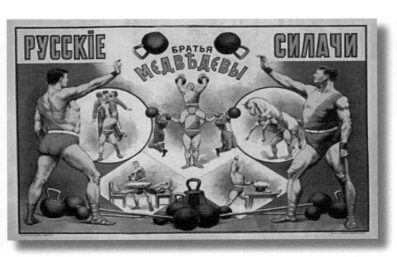

Kettlebells are compact, inexpensive, virtually indestructible, and can be used anywhere. The unique nature of kettlebell lifts provides a powerful training effect with a relatively light weight, and you can replace an entire gym with a couple of kettlebells. Dan John, Master SFG[1] and a highly accomplished power athlete, famously quipped, "With this kettlebell in my bedroom I can prepare myself for the Nationals."

Since I introduced the Russian kettlebell to the West in 1998, it has become a mainstay in the training of champions in sports ranging from powerlifting to MMA to triathlon. Elite special operations units have made the kettlebell an integral part of their training. They have discovered that kettlebells deliver extreme all-round fitness—and no single other tool does it better.

---

[1]SFG is the kettlebell education arm of my company StrongFirst. "G" stands for "girya."

Experience and science agree that kettlebell training develops a wide range of attributes: strength and power, various types of endurance, muscle hypertrophy, fat loss, health, and more. The kettlebell swing has been known to improve the deadlift of elite powerlifters—and the running times of high-level long distance runners. This is what gireviks call "the What the Hell Effect." The kettlebell defies the laws of specificity.

Russian kettlebell power to you!

SIMPLE & SINISTER

Competitive "sophistication" (rather, complication masked as sophistication) is harmful, as compared to the practitioner's craving for optimal simplicity.

—Nassim Nicholas Taleb, *Antifragile*

Simple & sinister.

Photo courtesy of U.S. military operator, name withheld

This program is as simple and sinister as the kettlebell itself.

I owe its name to a U.S. counterterrorist operator who used it to describe my system. I have been refining it ever since, making it even simpler while keeping it sinister.

In the XIV century, William of Occam of Occam's Razor fame gave the best training advice: "It is vain to do with more what can be done with less." The Simple & Sinister program (S&S) has been ruthlessly pruned down to only two exercises, known to deliver the widest range of benefits while being simple to learn and safe when properly executed. The programming is foolproof.

"IT IS VAIN TO DO WITH MORE WHAT CAN BE DONE WITH LESS."

Simple & Sinister is what Russians call a general preparation program.

- S&S will prepare you for almost anything life could throw at you, from carrying a piano upstairs to holding your own in a street fight.

- S&S will forge a fighter's physique, because the form must follow the function.

- S&S will give you the strength, the stamina, and the suppleness to recreationally play any sport—and play it well.

- If you are a serious athlete, S&S will serve as a perfect foundation for your sport-specific training.

- If you are a serious lifter, S&S will build your strength, rather than interfere with it.

Simple & Sinister will achieve all of the above while leaving plenty of time and energy to do your duty, your job, practice your sport, and have a life.

What S&S is not.

This is not a program to maximize any one attribute or performance in a particular event. If your goal is to press the heaviest kettlebell possible, to do 1,000 swings non-stop, to deadlift a record weight, or to win a championship race, S&S is not what you are looking for. That is what specialist programs are for—and they should always come after a foundation of general physical preparation has been laid. Otherwise you will only see short-term gains, you will fail to reach your potential, you might get hurt.

The majority of people, with the exception of competitive athletes at or above the high-intermediate level, do not need specialized training of that sort, and will get the most benefits with the least investment of time and energy from a powerful generalist program like S&S.

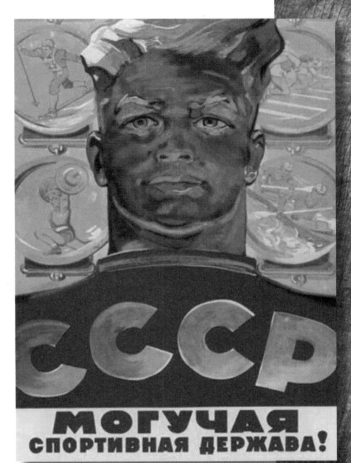

Here is the S&S plan in a nutshell.

There are only two moving parts, the swing and the get-up. No other exercises offer as many all-around benefits in such a tight package. "To build a superman, slow movements and quick lifts are required," taught Bob Hoffman of York Barbell. The get-up is the ultimate slow lift; the swing is the ultimate quick lift. The Yin and the Yang, both bases covered.

"TO BUILD A SUPERMAN, SLOW MOVEMENTS AND QUICK LIFTS ARE REQUIRED."

Andrey Kochergin, a Russian Special Forces vet and full contact karate master, likes to use Asian terminology to classify different types of breathing and muscular contractions. He explains that Yin breathing is used during wrestling, grappling, footwork, and some blocks. It is a steady, even breathing, punctuated by forced diaphragmatic exhalations during exertions. This describes the kettlebell get-up to a "t".

Yang breathing is breathing during a strike or some other explosive action. "A sharp exhalation is performed with maximal tension and ideally, for greater concentration, with a scream," comments Kochergin. "In the end of a Yang exhalation there is a breath hold, essential for instant concentration of a strike but counterproductive in long strength efforts of wrestling." This is the hard style kettlebell swing.

Mark Reifkind, Master SFG, calls the swing the most beneficial exercise anyone can do. Among its many benefits are superior conditioning, rapid fat loss, explosive hip power, killer grip, various back health benefits, and it is very easy on the knees. Rif adds that the swing is "scalable to a 70-year-old grandmother and to a 20-year-old super athlete."

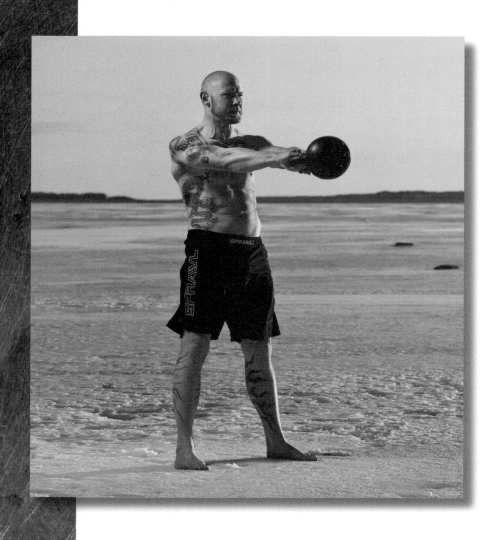

Arctic swings by Senior SFG Tommy Blom from Sweden.

Photo courtesy of Tommy Blom

The get-up is an old-time strongman stunt that is the king of "functional training." While everyone pays FT a lip service, the get-up delivers. When done with sufficient weight, it teaches the body many movement lessons that cannot be learned through sissy exercises with balls, bands, and Ken and Barbie dumbbells. Once you have conquered the get-up, you will be the master of your body, not its guest.

The get-up does magic for one's shoulders, making them remarkably resilient against Brazilian jiu-jitsu arm bars and heavy bench presses. The get-up is also one of the best ab exercises. Together with the swing, the get-up develops impressive, although not exaggerated, back and shoulders.

You will be training three to six times a week on a flexible schedule. Your workout is 100 swings total and five get-ups per arm, which is a very modest volume. Ivan Ivanov, formerly a coach for the Bulgarian National Gymnastics Team, noted: "A workout should give you more than it takes out of you."

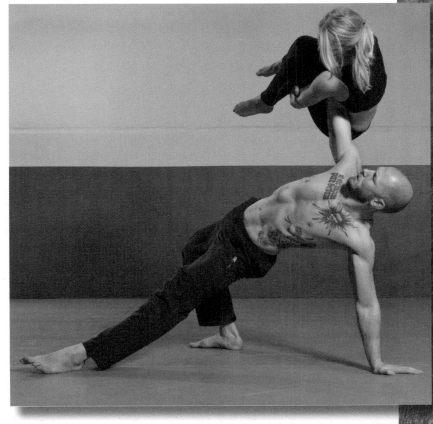

The human get-up. Do not try it at home.

Photo courtesy of Tommy Blom

"A WORKOUT SHOULD GIVE YOU MORE THAN IT TAKES OUT OF YOU."

You will be doing swings in sets of ten and get-ups in sets of one to assure the highest power output in swings and perfect technique in both. You will not be rushing between sets because the program is biased towards strength and quality.

S&S will leave gas in your tank for emergencies. A friend once wrote from down range, "Going hunting later today before dinner. A quick observation: The smart and most badass tactical athletes I see on a daily basis work hard, but always leave something in the tank. They owe their lives and those of their brothers to the ability to go hard every day and not be too sore from a workout."

Every two weeks you will test your readiness and your spirit, and push the pedal to the metal with a non-stop, all-out set of swings.

YOU ONLY NEED A FEW KETTLEBELLS

You can pry my kettlebell out of my dead cold hand.

—Anonymous

To paraphrase an ad for a Swiss watch, "You never really own a kettlebell. You merely look after it for the next generation." If you get quality bells and take care of them, they will outlive you. You might as well get good ones.

Russian kettlebells are traditionally measured in poods. One *pood*, an old Russian unit, equals 16 kilograms, approximately 35 pounds. For the S&S program, you need the following bell sizes.

The Kettlebells You Need

	Need right now	Will need soon
Average strength lady	18, 26, 35 lbs.	44, 53 lbs.
Strong lady	26, 35, 44 lbs.	53 lbs.
Average strength gentleman	35, 53 lbs.	70 lbs.
Strong gentleman	53, 70 lbs.	

Ladies, you need more bells because you have a different upper to lower body strength ratio than gents. You will see a discrepancy between the genders in the swing and get-up goals for the same reason.

Gireviks do not talk pounds, even in the US and the UK, so start memorizing your kettlebell weights in kilos. Here is the same chart in kilos.

	Need right now	Will need soon
Average strength lady	8, 12, 16kg	20, 24kg
Strong lady	12, 16, 20kg	24kg
Average strength gentleman	16, 24kg	32kg
Strong gentleman	24, 32kg	

If you are wondering what "strong" is, it is probably not you.

Your goal, eventually, is to dominate 35-pound get-ups and 53-pound one-arm swings if you are a lady—a 70-pounder for both lifts if you are a gentleman. Experience shows these numbers to be very achievable, and reaching them makes a dramatic difference in all-around fitness and body composition.

Should you decide to go beyond that, the ladies' goal is get-ups with 53 pounds and one-arm swings with 70 pounds. Gents get the 106-pound "Beast" for both drills.

Girevichkas: Lady Kettlebellers in Imperial Russia

In 1902 Linda "the Baltic Champion" Belling impressed the St. Petersburg Athletic Society by one-arm curling 32kg.

Agafiya Zavidnaya easily pressed a pair of 32s hanging on her pinkies well past her prime. Anna Geld, the wife of famous Russian clown Anatoly Durov, lifted heavy kettlebells and barbells on stage in the 1920s. To prove her strength was for real, Anna once challenged a male wrestler. She lost, but only after twenty minutes of ruthless fighting.

In 1913 circus performer Maria Lurs from Estonia juggled 32kg kettlebells and could one-arm snatch a three-pood—48kg! Ivan Lebedev wrote about her, "Every stunt of hers is full of strength, yet Maria Lurs' figure is not at all rough but amazes with its soft and supple lines... city ladies should see this Eve's daughter, rightfully proud of her strength and the harmony of her shape."

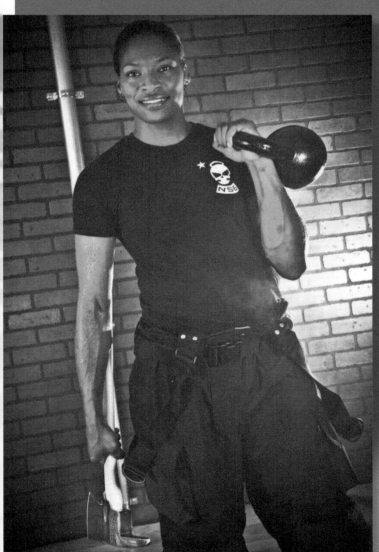

But don't get the idea the Russian city ladies were wimps. *St. Petersburg Gazette* reported in 1897, "The strongest of the lady athletes in our capital is Ms. M.S.P.... In spite of her young age and her 3-pood bodyweight she one-arm presses two poods and ten pounds... The second strongest has to be Mrs. E.G... It is interesting that this athlete is married and her husband is much weaker than her."

Take note, ladies. It can be done, especially in this age of feminized men. Pick up that kettlebell and you should have no trouble becoming a better man than most men.

A XXI century girevichka. Firefighter and SFG Team Leader Asha Wagner can do a strict pullup—dead hang, no kipping, neck to the bar—with a 70-pound kettlebell.

Photo courtesy of Asha Wagner

You might be surprised at the large jumps between sizes. The original intention was probably as mundane as saving roubles and square meters of storage space. Much later Soviet scientists like Prof. Arkady Vorobyev, also a weightlifting world and Olympic champion, discovered that sharp changes in load are superior to small changes when it comes to delivering the message to your body: "Get strong!"

There are other reasons for large jumps between weights. Dan John, Master SFG explains:

> Why I like kettlebells: I have so little choice. Dumbbells in many gyms go up by ten pounds, some five, some even a pound at a time. A thousand machines for bench presses... a million combos.
>
> Stop! The brain can only take so much!
>
> With kettlebells, I really have only up to three choices for an exercise... often only one.
>
> Less choice, less mental RAM going out the door. The more you choose, the less you have left to push the workout. Those leg innie and outie machines can convince you you're working your legs. You're not... but you can use your brain to convince you that you are.
>
> No choice. More work.

RESPECT YOUR KETTLEBELL

Once a year even an unloaded gun shoots.

—Russian range masters' observation

Kettlebells do not hurt people. People do.

A kettlebell will get your respect—the easy way or the hard way.

Here is the easy way.

1. **Get a medical clearance.**

    Get clearance, especially from an orthopedist and a cardiologist. The latter is no joking matter, since kettlebell training can be extremely intense.

2. **Always be aware of your surroundings.**

    Find a training area with a non-slippery surface on which you are not afraid to drop a kettlebell.

    The area must be clear of objects you might trip over—including other kettlebells—or that you might hit with a kettlebell. There should be no people or animals in a radius where you could injure them.

    Note the direction of the sun if you are practicing the get-up outdoors. Beware of getting dizzy from looking up toward the sky.

3. **Train barefoot or wear shoes with a flat, thin sole and room for the toes to spread.**

    Training barefoot is superior for health and performance reasons. If you must wear shoes, wear Converse Chuck Taylors, Vibram Five Fingers, or similar shoes that have thin soles and do not pinch the toes together. You have sensory receptors on the bottoms of your feet that make you stronger and improve balance and coordination. Wearing traditional shoes diminishes the ability of these receptors to work properly, and therefore impedes performance and can increase the risk of injury. Go native.

4. **Never contest for space with a kettlebell.**

    Do not try to save a rep that has gone wrong. Guide the kettlebell to fall harmlessly, and move out of the way if necessary. And remember, quick feet are happy feet.

5. **Practice all safety measures at all times.**

    Respect every kettlebell, even the lightest one. Always use perfect form picking up and setting down a kettlebell. The set is not over until the bell is safely parked.

6. **Keep moving once your heart rate is high.**

    After a hard set, keep moving by walking, shadow boxing, or moving your arms to help your heart pump the blood. Stop only when your heart rate is halfway down to normal. Consider getting a heart rate monitor.

7. **Don't put your spine into flexion during or after training.**

    Forward-bending stretches and slouching after training, harmless as these seem, could injure your back.

    Unless counter-indicated, back-bending stretches are recommended following training.

8. **Focus on quality, not quantity.**

    Gray Cook, physical therapist extraordinaire, points out that motor control goes south with fatigue and "the body will always sacrifice quality for quantity." When you are no longer able to continue with perfect technique, the gig is up.

Instruction cannot cover all contingencies and there is no substitute for good judgment. Be a responsible adult, not a victim.

BE A RESPONSIBLE ADULT, NOT A VICTIM.

TAKE THE BRAKES OFF YOUR STRENGTH

Flexibility gives me my strength. Flexibility is my weapon.

—Ichiro Suzuki, New York Yankees

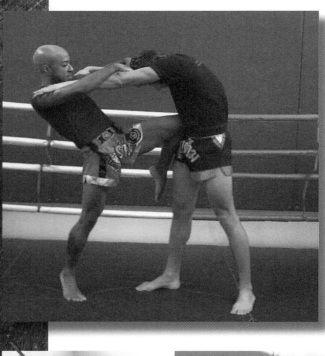

Strength that fails to reach is impotent.

Consider a Thai boxer throwing a vicious forward knee. The rear hip extends and the glute fully contracts and throws the whole body of the fighter into the strike—while adding a couple of inches of reach.

Now watch what happens when a character with tight hips tries to knee his opponent.

At StrongFirst we do not stretch just for the heck of it. We stretch to remove the brakes that prevent us from fully expressing our strength.

The three drills in this section have been cherry-picked to do just that.

The first exercise—the prying goblet squat—unlocks the pelvis and hips. The freedom of movement it will give you is mind-boggling.

The second exercise—the StrongFirst hip bridge—will stretch the hip flexors, the muscles on the top of the thighs that act like brakes for the glutes. It will release deadly strikes, fast sprints, and powerful jumps.

The third exercise—the halo—will stretch the upper back and shoulders to free your arms.

Start each practice with three circuits of five reps of each exercise.

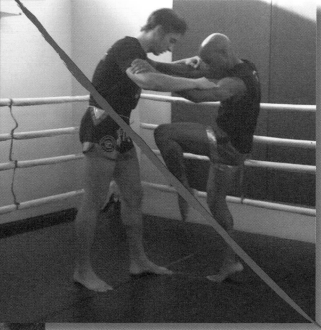

Cornell Ward and Gaius Ebratt, champion fighters coached by Steve Milles, SFG II.

Photos courtesy of Steve Milles of Five Points Academy, NYC

Prying Goblet Squat

I do not come from a culture where people are comfortable enough with the squat to make it the preferred resting position. But Russians do get enough squatting practice to maintain this fundamental movement pattern. Simple and sinister toilets (a hole in the floor) on the farms, in the military, at train stations, and many other places take care of that.

Americans and other Westerners need help. Enter the brilliantly simple goblet squat solution by Dan John, Master SFG. It is an exceptional stretch, especially the prying version.

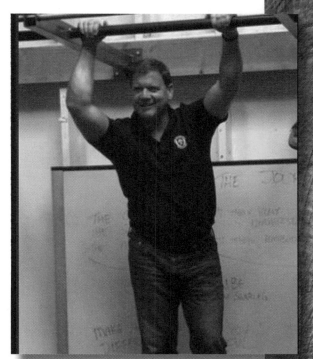

Dan John, Master SFG.

Photo courtesy of Dan John

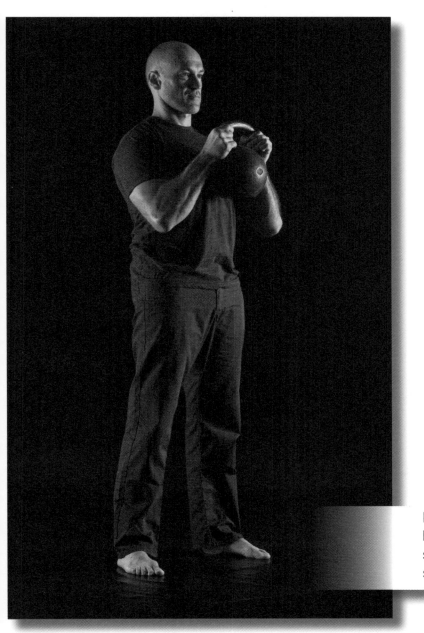

Do the drill barefoot. Pick up a light kettlebell by the horns and assume a shoulder-width stance with your feet slightly turned out.

11

Start the squat descent by pushing the knees apart.

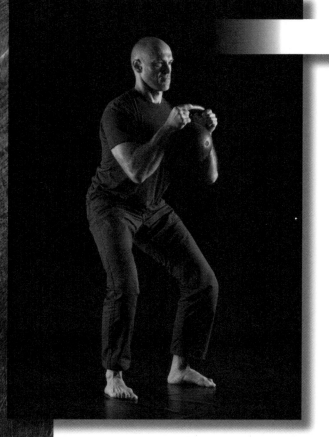

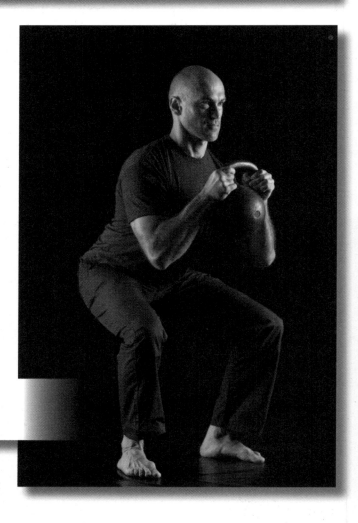

Do not drop straight down, but sit back slightly, to five o'clock, as if aiming to sit on a curb.

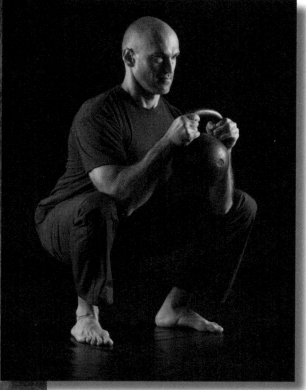

Do not allow your heels to come up. Go as deep as you can without pain.

Wedge your elbows inside your knees—exactly against the inner quads.

Push your knees apart with your elbows—without letting your big toes and the balls of the feet come off the ground.

Stay on the bottom of the squat. Relax without letting the spine round. Keep your chest up and stay tall without tilting your head back. Do not shrug your shoulders—just the opposite. Breathe in a relaxed manner.

Start "prying" your hips loose. I use this verb literally. Imagine pulling a massive wooden post out of the ground. Pulling straight up will do very little, unless your name is King Kong or Eddie Coan. You will have to pry the post back and forth and side to side.

You are going to do this prying with your hips. There are two goals. One is to separate your pelvis into two halves, to "widen" it. Mobilizing your pelvis may spare you from many orthopedic problems down the road. Two, the idea is to pull the hip joints out of their sockets. Do not panic—it is just a visualization. Unless you are hypermobile, it would take Alexander Karelin's best efforts to dislocate your hips.

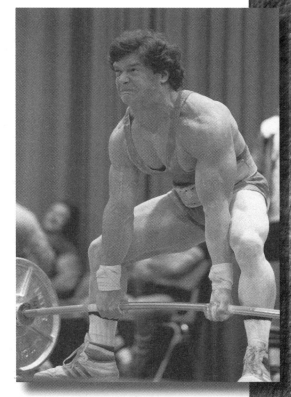

Powerlifting legend Ed Coan:
"Only the weak need to pry."

Photo courtesy of Powerlifting USA

With this in mind, move your pelvis in different directions.

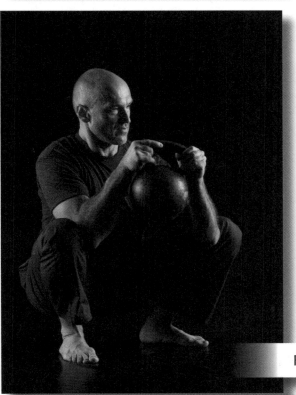

Make space.

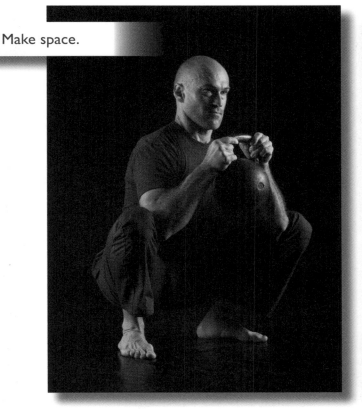

Pull your hip joints out of their sockets.

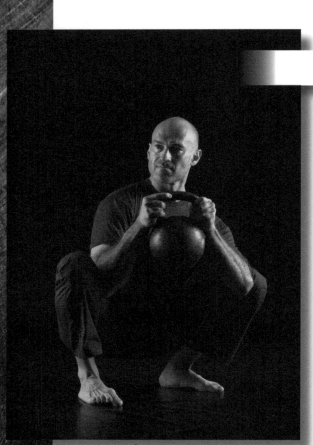

Make your pelvis wider.

This is a good time to shuffle around and adjust your stance; remember where that stance is next time you squat.

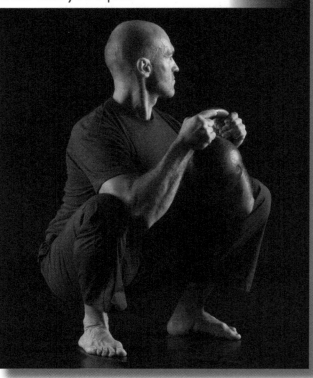

Your pelvis will keep sinking. Go as deep as you can without flexing your spine or experiencing pain. Do not allow the elbows to drop.

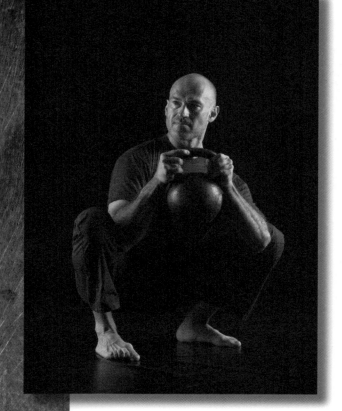

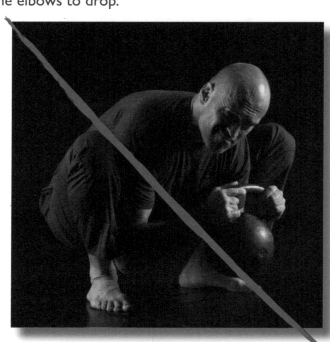

14

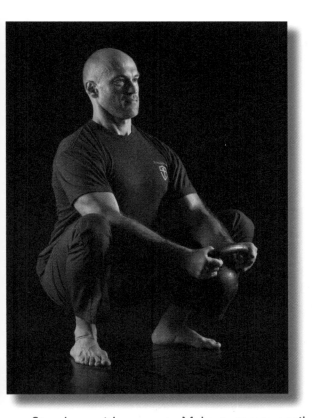

Do a few curls without moving the elbows—seriously. It is a form of prying: the moving kettlebell shifts the center of gravity back and forth. Jack Reape, an American record holder in the bench press, was caught doing this at a gym. Admiring Jack's pipes, the kid asked if this was his favorite biceps exercise. Deadpan, Jack replied, "Favorite and only."

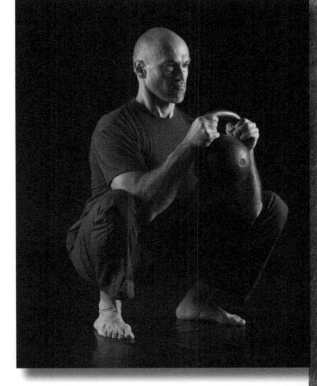

Stand up with a grunt. Make sure your tail does not rise faster than your head. Lock your knees and contract the glutes at the top.

If you are too weak to stand up with good form, sit back on the floor and park the bell.

Do five reps, resting between them if necessary.

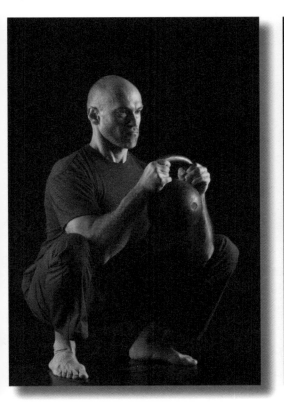

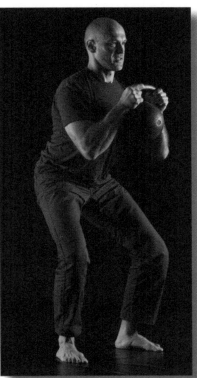

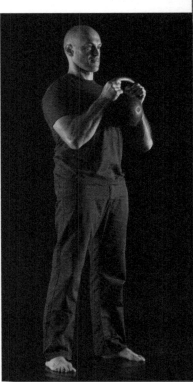

StrongFirst Hip Bridge

Lie on your back with your feet flat and knees bent about ninety degrees, as if you are about to do crunches.

Squeeze a pair of cushy shoes—the kind I do not recommend for lifting—between your knees. This will force you to extend your hips instead of overarching the lower back. Grip the ground with your toes, dig your heels in, and lift the pelvis as high as possible. Pause for three seconds, constantly trying to lift higher and higher, then come down and relax. Rest briefly, and repeat. Do five reps in this manner.

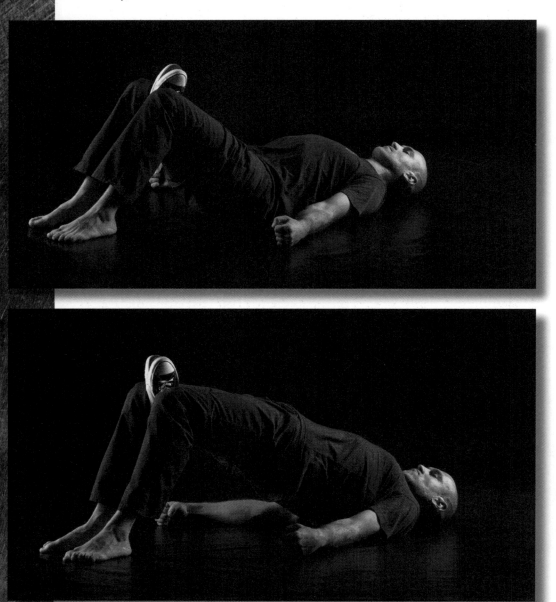

I must stress this point: This is not a muscular endurance exercise. Your job is not to see how long you can hold the bridge, but to get the maximal glute contraction and the greatest range of motion. Drive your pelvis through, as the fighter in the picture on page ten. Not fast, but strong. The goal is for the pelvis to rise high enough for the thighs to form a straight line with the torso.

If you are a martial artist, humor me and throw a couple of front knees or kicks against a target right after these. You will see a big difference in reach and power.

Halo

This drill by Steve Maxwell is very simple, yet it covers many bases of upper-body mobility.

Hold a light kettlebell upside down by its horns or grab a light barbell plate. Lock your knees. Tense the glutes to protect your back.

Keeping your shoulders down as much as possible, slowly circle the bell or plate around your head, progressively tighter and lower.

Five circles in both directions are about right.

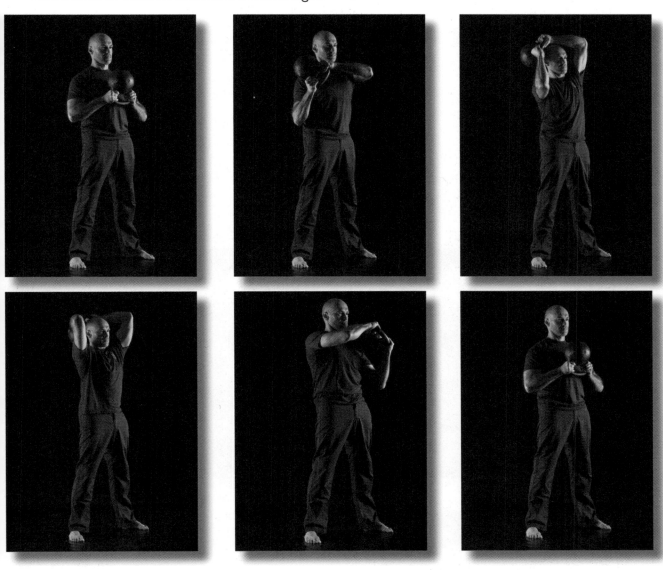

Perform the above three drills in the specified order for three circuits before your kettlebell training. The above regimen is meant to bring a moderately tight but healthy person up to speed. You might have some issues that need to be resolved with the help of a medical professional and later a certified SFG kettlebell instructor.[2]

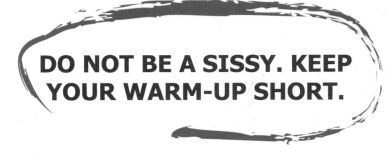

DO NOT BE A SISSY. KEEP YOUR WARM-UP SHORT.

[2]You will find our international certified instructor directory at www.strongfirst.com/instructors/

If you have a medical condition, follow the warm-up advice of your medical professional. If you do not have a condition, do not be a sissy and keep it short.

Right after the S&S sessions, or later, preferably shortly before bedtime, do the following relaxed stretches for the hip area so heavily involved in both swings and get-ups. Do one to three sets of each in a circuit.

90/90 Stretch

Explains Dr. Michael Hartle, Master SFG:

> This modified hurdler stretch is great for the hips and lower back. It stretches the gluteus muscles and the various hip rotators. Sit on the floor on your left hip. Place your left leg, bent at a right angle, in front of you, and your right leg, bent at a right angle, to the side. The starting position will have right angles at both the right and left hip, knee and ankle, with the left foot parallel to the right calf and the left calf parallel to the right thigh.
>
> Place your right hand on your left ankle and your left hand, with the left arm rotated out, on the ground outside your left hip. Making a "proud chest" and hinging at the hips only (no rounding the spine!), lean forward and press your buttocks away, keeping the sternum over the knee. Hold the stretch… making sure to relax and breathe deeply. Keep the neck and head in line with the torso. Repeat on the opposite side.

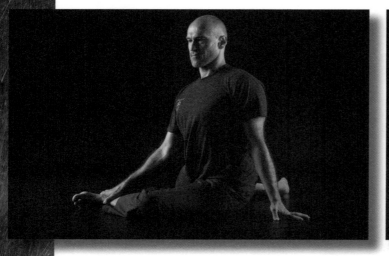 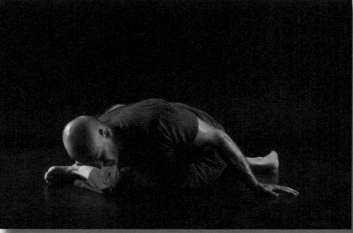

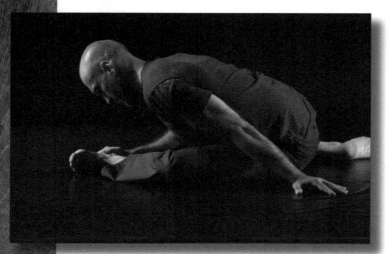

Diagonally turning your upper body towards the front foot and repeating the directions above will provide an additional stretch for this area. When performed properly, this stretch will be felt in the outside of the front hip.

QL Straddle

This stretch is for the sides of the back. Sit in a straddle position. Do not open too wide, even if you can. A near split will shift the focus of the stretch elsewhere.

You are about to stretch your right side by reaching towards the left. Stretch your right arm overhead and get "tall."

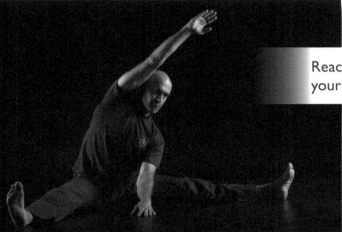

Reach forward—perpendicular to your left leg—with your left arm. Anchor your fingertips on the ground.

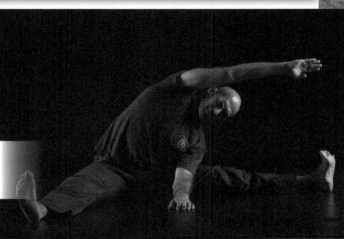

Lean to the left, reaching over your head with the right arm.

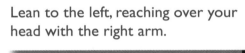

Breathe and relax. Gradually reach farther and farther, hopefully far enough to grab your toes. If you are tight, holding on to a bungee cord attached to a stationary object will help.

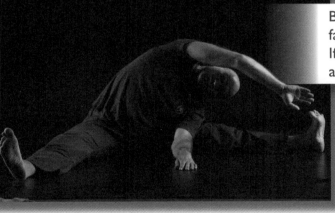

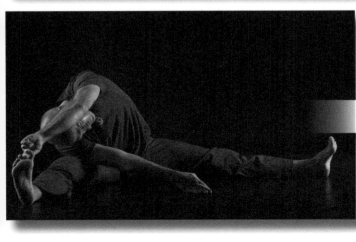

Repeat on both sides, naturally.

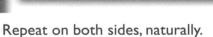

Nothing will happen in a single minute. The longer you stay in these two stretches and breathe through the tight spots, the better.

THE MOST POWERFUL HUMAN MOVEMENT

The hip hinge is the most powerful movement a human can do. It's the apex movement of an apex hunter!

—Dan John

A swing is not a squat.

A swing is a pull or hip hinge, in the same category as the deadlift, clean, and snatch, whether kettlebell or barbell.

Here is the difference. In a squat the knees and the hips flex to a similar degree on the way down. In a pull the hips do most of the flexion.

In both pulls and squats, the spine stays neutral.

IN A SQUAT THE KNEES AND THE HIPS FLEX TO A SIMILAR DEGREE ON THE WAY DOWN. IN A PULL THE HIPS DO MOST OF THE FLEXION.

Hip Hinge

You are about to learn to hinge through the hips.

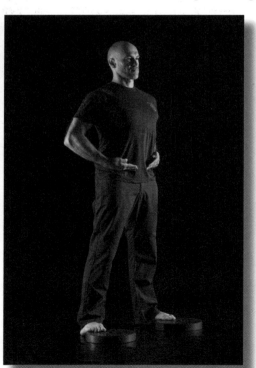

Stand with your feet slightly wider than your shoulders—wide enough to safely swing a large kettlebell between the knees. Turn your toes slightly outward, a lot less than forty-five degrees. Elevate your toes and the balls of the feet on 2x4s, 25-pound barbell plates, thick books, or other flat, equal-height objects. This tactic will prevent you from cheating because it stops the knees from slipping forward.

Open your chest and place the outside edges of your hands into the creases at the top of your thighs. Shift your weight to your heels and chop your hands hard into your hip "hinges" to push the pelvis back. Feel the muscles in the hip creases contracting as you hinge.

Your knees and ankles will naturally flex somewhat, but not to the point of losing a stretch in the hamstrings. Focus on folding at the hips.

In all of the deadlift and swing evolutions, you must track the toes with the knees. In other words, push the knees slightly out to prevent them from collapsing in.

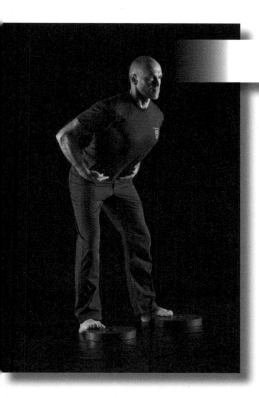

Push your tail back as far as you can—*back, not down.*

Look at the horizon for the duration of the drill. Keep your head up without jamming your neck.

Hinge as far as you can without rounding your back.

A SWING IS NOT A SQUAT. A SWING IS A PULL OR HIP HINGE.

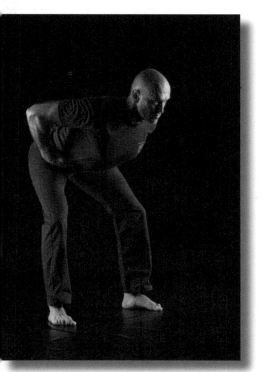

Stand up by contracting your glutes—"crush a walnut."

Practice the hip hinge until it becomes crisp and automatic. Then remove the crutches of the 2x4s, but pretend they are still there, forcing the shins to stay near-vertical. The knees may slightly move—but no farther than the mid-foot. It is the only way to maintain a powerful bow-like stretch of the hamstrings.

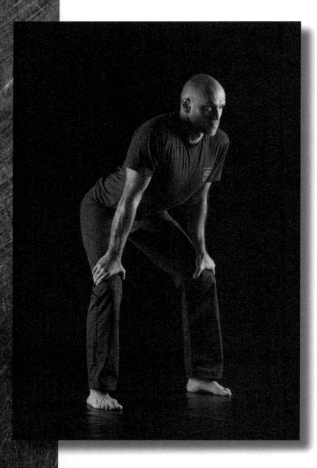

Short-Stop Drill

Prof. Stuart McGill's short-stop drill will teach you other essential elements of professional deadlift and swing technique.

Assume the hip-hinge stance and hinge through your hips. Strongly grab your thigh muscles above the kneecaps. Lock your elbows, then shift your weight slightly towards your heels.

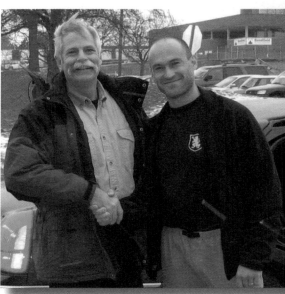

Prof. McGill with the author.

Photo courtesy of Prof. Stuart McGill's Spine Biomechanics Lab, University of Waterloo, Canada

Stuart McGill, the world's leading spine biomechanist, comments: "Enjoy carrying the weight of your upper body down the arms and onto the thighs. Focus on the curves in your torso—are they the same as when you were standing? If they are, you have good form. If they are not, adjust them back to the natural curves."

Now "anti-shrug" your shoulders with your lats. This is extremely important. At StrongFirst we call the lats the "super muscles." Engaged properly, they help protect the spine and shoulders and increase strength in lower- and upper-body exercises. Push down hard with your armpits while pushing the chest out.

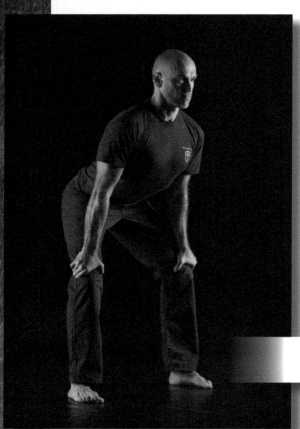

You are in a very powerful posture and it should feel like it.

You know how to stand up: Contract your glutes and drive your pelvis forward.

Deadlift

Straddle a kettlebell between your heels. Parking it farther behind you will activate your lats even more, and teach you valuable skills for the swing.

Take a breath and force your shoulders down away from your ears—the anti-shrug.

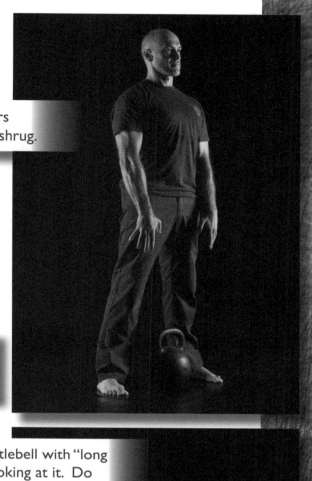

Sit back, loading your heels, but not letting the toes come off the ground.

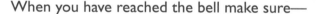

Reach for the kettlebell with "long arms" without looking at it. Do not lose the lat contraction and the anti-shrug; do not allow your upper back and chest to collapse.

When you have reached the bell make sure—

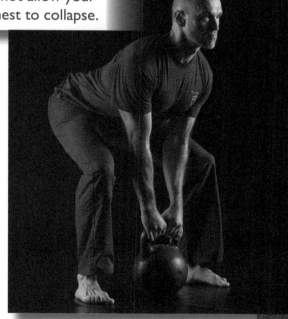

- the lower back is flat or slightly arched. *(If you cannot help rounding because your hamstrings are tight, temporarily elevate the kettlebell on a box or a few books and work on your flexibility.)*

- the chest is open, the head is up and the eyes are on the horizon.

- the shoulders are pressed down, away from the head—anti-shrug.

- the weight is slightly towards the heels.

- the shins are nearly vertical; the knees may not be farther forward than the mid-foot. *(You may bring back the 2x4s if you are having trouble.)*

- the pelvis is higher than the knees, but lower than the shoulders.

- the arms are straight.

- the knees are tracking the toes.

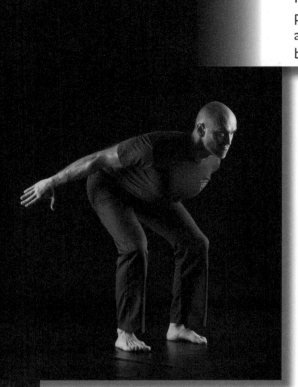

If you brought your feet closer together, the bottom position would look exactly like the bottom of a natural athlete's standing broad jump, power-coiled in every lower-body muscle.

THE DEADLIFT IS THE ULTIMATE EXPRESSION OF FULL-BODY POWER —LIKE A JUMP.

Hook the kettlebell handle with your fingers, but do not grip it tightly. Take the slack out of your armpits. You are ready to stand up.

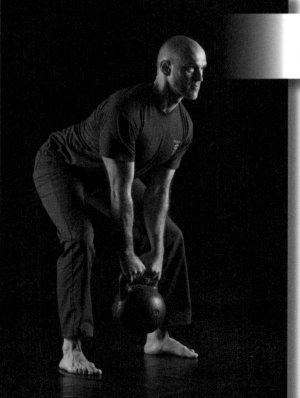

Stand up ramrod straight—snappy, although not quite explosive.

Your pelvis must never rise faster than your shoulders. Marty Gallagher teaches: "Everything must arrive at once." You want everything to travel as one piece—as in a jump.

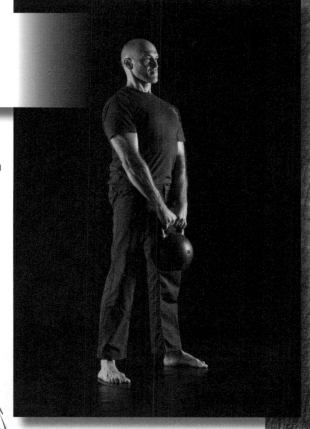

At the lockout your body must form a straight line. The knees are locked, the back and neck are neutral. Do not lean back; imagine standing with your back flush against a wall.

Tense every muscle below your neck—*plank*. Pull up the kneecaps. Cramp the glutes. Brace the abs, as if you are about to be punched. Keep the lats locked and loaded. You are a board.

BRACING MEANS TIGHTENING UP YOUR ABS AS IF YOU ARE ABOUT TO GET PUNCHED—IT DOES NOT MEAN SUCKING IN YOUR STOMACH!

At the same time, keep your traps relaxed and your face impassive.

Pause for an instant, and then start the descent by hinging back. Maintain perfect form and do not be concerned with the speed of the movement.

Without looking at the kettlebell, touch it to the ground between your heels. The kettlebell will begin to land in front of you. Do not let it. Guide it back with your lats—*"swim"* it back.

Although traditionally deadlifts are done with a pause on the platform between reps—hence the original name of the "dead weight lift"—for our purposes touch-and-go deads are optimal. As soon as you touch the deck, immediately stand up.

Inhale through your nose on the way down; forcefully but not completely exhale on the way up.

Practice in sets of five to ten reps, always ending with the kettlebell between your heels. Do not use a mirror, but I strongly encourage you to film yourself for review.

THE SWING -- A FAT-BURNING ATHLETE-BUILDER*

Kettlebell high-rep ballistics are the closest you can get to fighting without throwing a punch.

—A federal counterterrorist operator

The swing is a Russian army knife of exercises. What else do you call an exercise that can increase both a professional powerlifter's strength and an elite marathoner's endurance?

"The Swing is The Thing," states Rif. "It's the best exercise for almost everyone—beginners to elite athletes, youngsters to the elders. I just can't find another exercise that is as easy on the body and makes one work as hard as the hard style kettlebell swing. It strengthens the body at the same time it heals it."

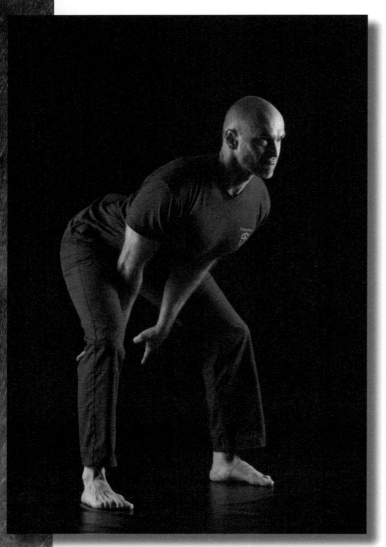

Hike Pass

The top of the swing is a plank. The bottom is what Dan John calls the "silverback" stance.

Assume the bottom position of the deadlift—without the kettlebell. Press your straight arms against your body—the upper arms against the ribs and the forearms against the upper inner thighs—high up. The more snugly your arms are pressed against your legs and torso, the more powerful the swings will be. You will be literally launching the bell with your body, as opposed to waiting for the power to be transmitted through the shoulders.

Now stretch your fingertips and sternum as far apart as you can. Reach back with the former, and forward with the latter. Remember this stretched and loaded sensation and note where your hands and thus the kettlebell would be. This is where you will actively guide the bell to from now on.

* The title of this chapter is a quote from Dan John.

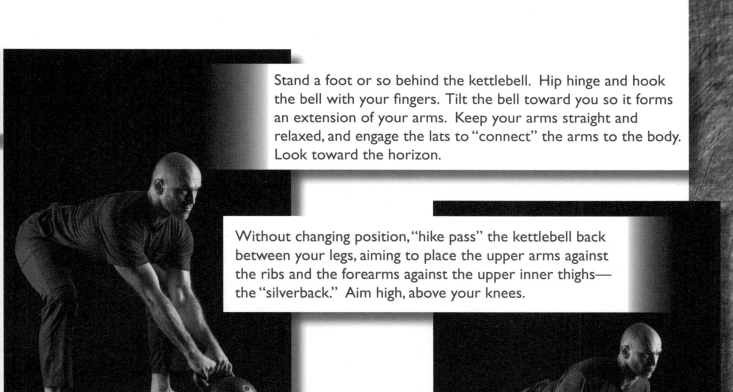

Stand a foot or so behind the kettlebell. Hip hinge and hook the bell with your fingers. Tilt the bell toward you so it forms an extension of your arms. Keep your arms straight and relaxed, and engage the lats to "connect" the arms to the body. Look toward the horizon.

Without changing position, "hike pass" the kettlebell back between your legs, aiming to place the upper arms against the ribs and the forearms against the upper inner thighs— the "silverback." Aim high, above your knees.

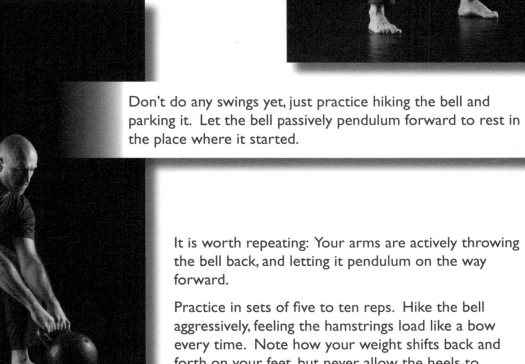

Don't do any swings yet, just practice hiking the bell and parking it. Let the bell passively pendulum forward to rest in the place where it started.

It is worth repeating: Your arms are actively throwing the bell back, and letting it pendulum on the way forward.

Practice in sets of five to ten reps. Hike the bell aggressively, feeling the hamstrings load like a bow every time. Note how your weight shifts back and forth on your feet, but never allow the heels to unload.

Two-Arm Swing

When you have the hike pass down, start swinging. Hike and pendulum the bell for a few reps and then, once you find a rhythm, explosively straighten after finishing a hike pass. Look at the horizon for the duration of the drill. Keep your head up without jamming your neck.

As before, do not think about the bell on the way up. Drive with your hips and let it freely pendulum. On the upswing the arms and shoulders only transfer the hips' power, but they do not lift the kettlebell. The arms must be straight and loose to do the job—like ropes. If your technique is correct, the kettlebell will form an extension of the arms.

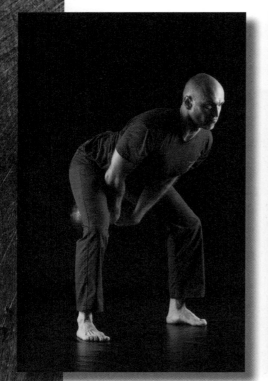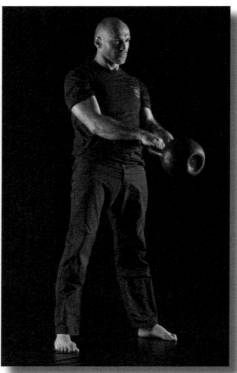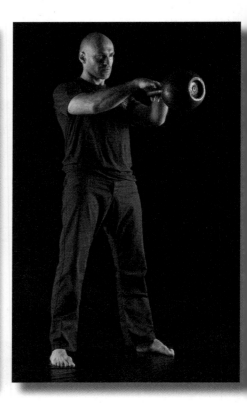

Memorize this: *In the swing the arms work on the negative, the hips on the positive.*

IN THE SWING THE ARMS WORK ON THE NEGATIVE, THE HIPS ON THE POSITIVE.

If you are doing everything right, the bell will naturally go up to a level somewhere between your stomach and shoulders. Do not try to swing it higher! Like a broad jump or a straight punch, the swing is an exercise in projecting power forward.

On a related subject, do not lean back at the top of the swing. Let your glutes do the job; leave your back out of it. It is also very important to brace your abs.

If your heels come up, release the kettlebell to protect your back! This applies to all swing evolutions. Soon you will learn to play a tug-of-war with the kettlebell and subtly change the weight distribution on your feet in response to the kettlebell's shenanigans.

Incidentally, being able to reflexively react to such perturbations is an important component of back pain prevention—and research shows that kettlebell swings improve this ability.

In addition, you will increase agility and athletic power. "Balance boosts power," states Dr. Michael Colgan, explaining that it takes more energy to move an unbalanced body.

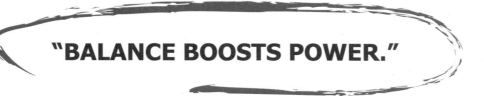

"BALANCE BOOSTS POWER."

After five to ten reps, park the kettlebell in front of you as you practiced in the hike pass and pendulum drills. Remember, until the kettlebell is safely parked, the set is not over! Keep practicing the swings. You no longer need to pendulum the bell for reps before swinging it—just one hike and go.

Be explosive. But do not confuse speed with panic.

DO NOT CONFUSE SPEED WITH PANIC.

Next work on your breathing. Forcefully exhale on the way up; sharply inhale through your nose on the way down. In the future when you are doing hard swing workouts, you will need to learn how to take two sharp inhalations back to back on the way down.

To help you find the breathing rhythm, loudly call out the number of each rep at the top of the swing. Loud. Louder!

Later, once you have fully dialed in the breathing rhythm, switch to grunts or *Tssa!!!* sounds. Do not try to be quiet; the swing is not that type of exercise. The swing is full of spirit, like a karate punch. *KIAI!!!*

Along with your battle cry, cramp your glutes, brace your abs, and pull up your kneecaps.

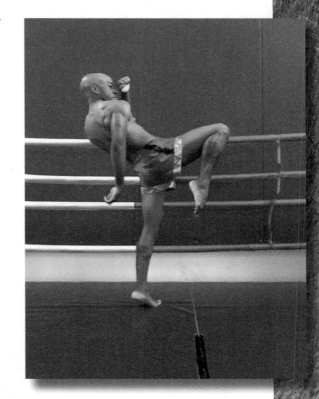

Drive your hips through!

Photo courtesy of Steve Milles of Five Points Academy

Here is a key subtlety to work on next: Once the kettlebell has reached the apex of its flight, let it float for an instant. Then, once it has started falling, guide it back between your legs using the lats. Stay upright and do not release the glutes until your forearms almost hit your stomach. At the very last instant, hinge your hips and get out of the way. Play chicken with the kettlebell.

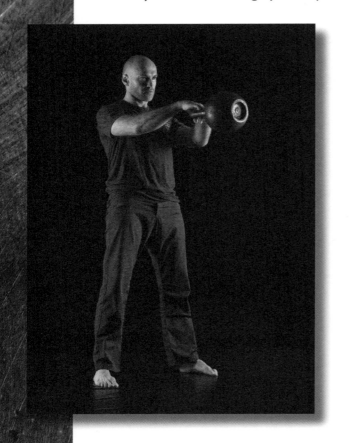 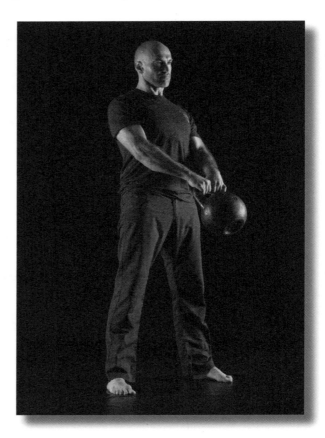

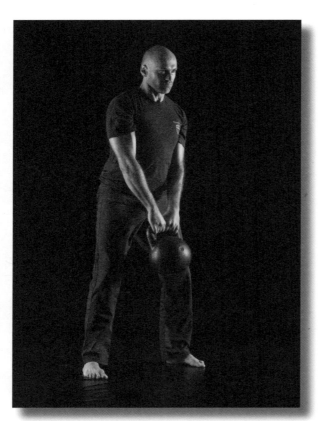 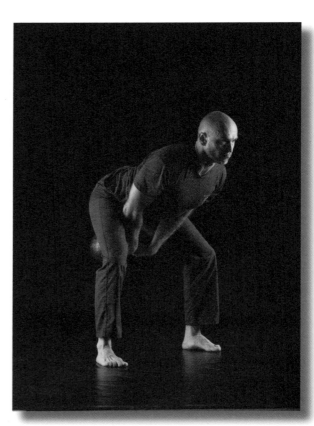

I must make a point here. A hard style swing demands maximally explosive individual reps—not maximum speed. Enjoy the float on the top; it is the only rest you are going to get.

A HARD STYLE SWING DEMANDS MAXIMALLY EXPLOSIVE INDIVIDUAL REPS —NOT MAXIMUM RPM.

One-Arm Swing

A passage in Nassim Nicholas Taleb's *Antifragile* caught my eye: "People who build strength using these modern expensive gym machines can lift extremely large weights, show great numbers and develop impressive-looking muscles, but fail to lift a stone; they get completely hammered in a street fight by someone trained in more disorderly settings. Their strength is extremely domain-specific and their domain doesn't exist outside."

"Disorderly settings" are what you need when you are after all-terrain strength.

Enter the one-arm swing. The bell not only pulls you forward, but it is determined to twist you as well. It is seriously "antifragile" when a man can show a 48kg who is the boss, or a woman a 32kg.

DISORDERLY SETTINGS ARE WHAT YOU NEED WHEN YOU ARE AFTER ALL-TERRAIN STRENGTH.

An asymmetrical load seriously challenges the stabilizers and increases the recruitment of many muscles. When I swung a 32kg kettlebell two-handed in Prof. Stuart McGill's lab, my glutes fired up to 80% maximal voluntary isometric contraction (MVC). When I did it one-handed, the recruitment was up to 100%. And the lat contraction jumped from 100% to 150%! In case you are wondering how it is possible to contract a muscle 150%, the max is isometric. In dynamic contractions higher values are possible—plyometrics are a case in point.

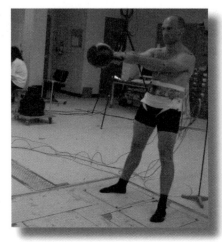 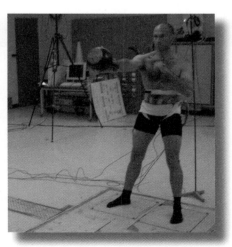

The swing on the left generates more power. The one on the right recruits more muscle.

Photos courtesy of Prof. Stuart McGill's Spine Biomechanics Lab, University of Waterloo, Canada

Last but not least, the one-arm swing is an exceptional grip-builder.

Why would you do two-arm swings at all if the one-arm version is so great? Because two-arm swings generate more power, as proven on the force platform. With reduced stabilization demands, you can really let it rip. Hence, do both types of swings.

When you are very competent in the two-arm swing, and not a moment sooner, add the one-arm swing to your practice.

One-Arm Swing Technique

Set the kettlebell on the floor with its handle parallel to your shoulders. With the working arm, loosely grip the handle in the middle—hook it with your fingers. Take the slack out of your shoulder using your lat.

Square your shoulders—more or less.

The hard style one-arm swing is an anti-rotation exercise. In other words, the weight is trying to twist you, while you insist on staying on a straight and narrow. That said, it is impossible to avoid some rotation, especially with a heavy bell—which is why I wrote more or less.

Now swing.

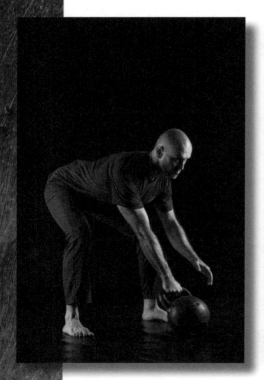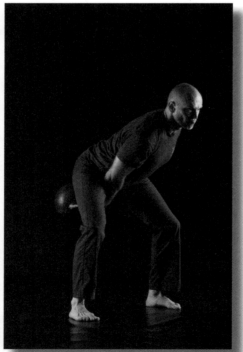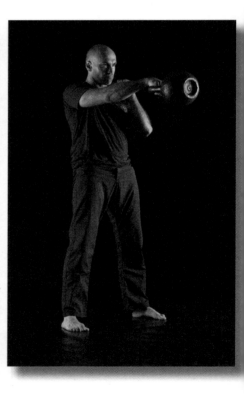

At the top of the rep, the kettlebell will surge forward, twisting your torso and pulling your shoulder out of its socket. Do not let it. Square your shoulders and pack the working shoulder. Packing refers to pulling the shoulder into its socket, the way a turtle retracts its head into its body. Do not shrug the shoulder up.

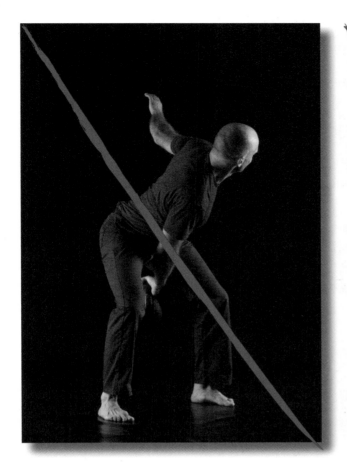
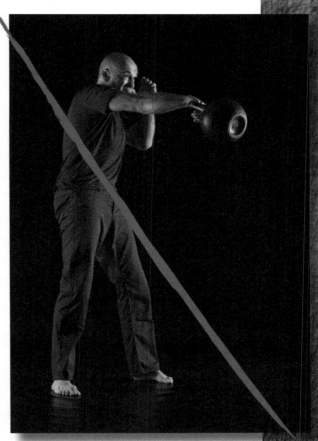

As for the free arm, let it naturally swing back on the way down. Do not overdo it to the point of making your spine twist. Let it swing up on the upswing to end in the on-guard position.

Hand-to-Hand Swing (H2H)

A squad of Russian soldiers has been digging a ditch for hours. Finally a young trooper makes the mistake of asking the squad leader when would they get to rest. "Rest when the dirt is in the air. The farther you throw it, the more rest you get," answers the sergeant.

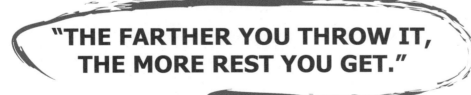

"THE FARTHER YOU THROW IT, THE MORE REST YOU GET."

This is also the secret to a great swing.

Maximally cramp the glutes and pop the hips to make the kettlebell weightless for an instant. Do not rush—let the bell float while keeping the glutes tight. All of your swings should be done this way, but the H2H version, which demands a hand switch on the fly, really drives home the point. Brett Jones, Master SFG, calls this "pop and float."

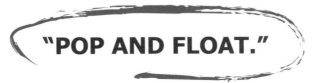

"POP AND FLOAT."

The second lesson the H2H swing teaches is "taming the arc." At the top of each rep, release the bell and catch it with the other hand. It will not want to cooperate. When an object is accelerating in an orbit, the centrifugal force pulls it away from the center. David took advantage of this force when he slayed Goliath with his sling.

You need to bring the bell in closer—"tame the arc," as Rob Lawrence put it. This is done by shrugging the shoulder back, not up—like starting a lawn mower. Do not pull with the biceps.

Pluck the bell out of the air with your other hand and carry on. If you have failed to tame the arc and the only way you can catch the bell is by reaching forward, abort. Let the bell fall and save your back to swing another day.

The H2H swing is not a part of the S&S plan because it is less challenging to the grip than the one-arm swing. It is just a drill to make two-arm and one-arm swings feel the same: *Pop and float, tame the arc.*

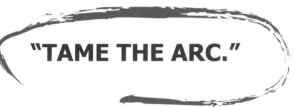
"TAME THE ARC."

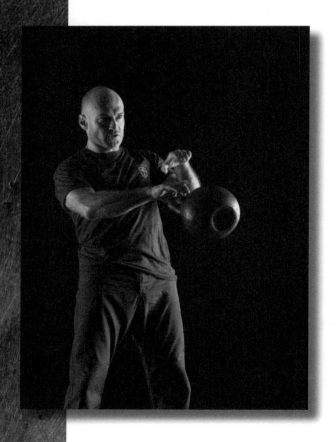
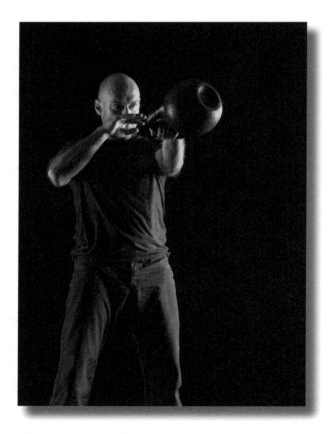

Take Care of Your Hands

Arm-wrestling is a blue collar sport. Competitors would not be caught dead moisturizing, exfoliating, and practicing other metrosexual nonsense. Marty, one of the best middleweights at our club, counted on this when he dropped his psych bomb. As soon as he gripped up with another puller but before the ref gave the *Go!* command, Marty opened his eyes wide and pronounced deadpan: "Your skin is so smooth and silky!" The other guy burst out laughing just as the "Go!" rang out. Laughter relaxes. Marty pinned his opponent in a flash.

That mind game would not have worked on a girevik. The manliest men of the kettlebell begrudgingly take care of their skin because bleeding calluses do not build character, and waste valuable training time. Here is how to avoid them.

Get quality kettlebells with smooth handles.

Gradually build up your training volume.

Do not abuse chalk—a little is good; a lot may make the skin tear.

Do not overgrip the bell in swings. Hook the handle with your fingers and try not to pinch the callusses at the bases of the fingers. As you get more skilled, you will find ways to rest the grip in certain phases of the swing, and regrip on the fly.

Moisturize your mitts before going to bed, hopefully with something manly like Cornhuskers Lotion.

Do not let calluses get thick. At night soak them in hot water and scrape them off with pumice stone. Don't scrape too thin though, just enough to get rid of the protruding parts that are likely to get pinched. Then do that "moisturizing" thing.

If it feels like a callus or blister is about to go, stop to swing another day.

Step-by-Step Blister Care
by Kristann Heinz, MD, SFG

1. When you first detect a blister, stop the activity. Do not break or pop the blister. The skin covering the blister helps to protect it from infection.

2. Gently wash with soap, or clean with Betadine if you are not near a sink. If the blister is broken, wash the area. If the blister came from kettlebell training, it is important to clean the blister of any paint or metal filings that may be imbedded in the blister area.

3. Next, apply antibiotic ointment such as Neosporin or Bacitracin to the area.

4. Protect the blister with a blister doughnut. You can buy moleskin at a drugstore. Cut out a circle of the moleskin slightly larger than the blister area. Place the moleskin ring around the blister.

5. Cover the blister area with gauze and secure it with hypoallergenic tape. This should reduce the friction to the area. Change the blister dressing daily.

6. With proper care a blister should heal in three to five days.

7. Monitor the healing. If you find the blister area is increasingly red, swollen, painful or you notice pus, the blister may be infected. Check to see if you have a fever.. The blister needs to be looked at by medical professional, who may prescribe antibiotics for a skin infection or cellulitis.

If you have a torn callus, follow these care instructions for a broken blister.

Do not let me catch you wearing those sissy gym gloves! Thin cotton gardening gloves with the fingers cut off are acceptable.

So are "sock sleeves," as suggested by Tracy "The Swing Queen" Reifkind, SFG. You will need a pair of medium thickness crew socks—new socks, since worn elastic will not hold the sleeves in place. Cut off the tops of the socks, about two inches wide, three if you have big hands. Center the sock sleeve on the callus line and you are ready for swings. You may use sock sleeves all the time or just for an occasional high-volume challenge. Do not wear them for get-ups.

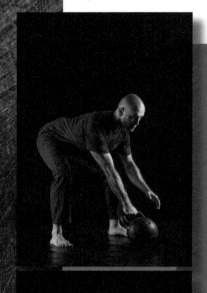

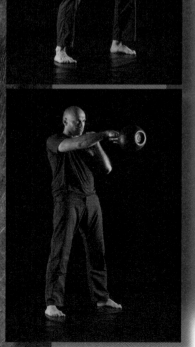

Swing Standards

Task:

Swing, one arm

Condition:

Swing a kettlebell back between your legs and then in front up to the chest level.

Standard:

1. The back is neutral. The neck is slightly extended or neutral on the bottom of the swing.

2. The heels, toes, and the balls of the feet are planted, and the knees track the toes.

3. The working shoulder is packed.

4. The kettlebell handle passes above the knees during the backswing.

5. The working arm is straight at the bottom position.

6. There is no forward knee movement on the upswing.

7. The body forms a straight line at the top of the swing. The hips and knees fully extend; the spine is neutral.

8. The kettlebell forms an extension of the forearm at the top of the swing; the arm is almost straight.

9. Inhale on the way down; forcefully exhale on the way up.

10. The abs and glutes visibly contract at the top of the swing.

11. The kettlebell floats for a second at the top of the swing.

THE GET-UP -- YOUR STRONGMAN MENTOR

The get-up is loaded yoga.

—Gray Cook

Legend has it that old-time strongmen taught apprentices the get-up and told them to come back when able to do it with 100 pounds.

The skills and strength the apprentice would acquire over the many months of pursuing this noble goal would be far superior to whatever a roomful of personal trainers could have produced during the same time—and no words would have been wasted.

The aspiring strongman would be repeating his childhood development process, in a way. Roll over... prop up... kneel... victoriously stand up. Wobbly in the beginning, he would gain confidence with every rep.

I was introduced to this exercise by Steve Maxwell. The get-up is at least 200 years old, and modern specialists view it as an exceptionally functional exercise. Gray Cook, physical therapist to Navy SEALs and NFL teams, said, "The Turkish get-up is the perfect example of training primitive movement patterns—from rolling over, to kneeling, to standing and reaching. If I were limited to choosing only one exercise, it would be the Turkish get-up."

When our strongman apprentice finally got to 70-100 pounds, his real learning would begin. "Heavy weight is instructive," states Cook. There is nothing like a big ball of iron overhead to teach you about physics. You will instinctively know you had better place your foot or hand *just so*—or else.

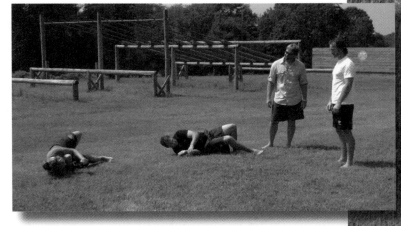

Gray Cook coaching the get-up.

Photo courtesy of Gray Cook

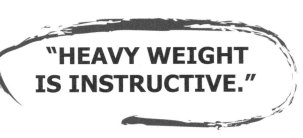

"HEAVY WEIGHT IS INSTRUCTIVE."

The apprentice would also learn that, in Dan John's words, "The body is one piece."

Many athletes never learn that crucial lesson—and never have a shot at a title. The get-up will be kind enough to explain it to you. Your abs will fire like crazy; peak activation in excess of 100% in all main midsection muscles has been documented in a get-up with only 50 pounds. Work up to a heavy weight in the get-up and your torso will be up to the standards of Ron Swanson's Pyramid of Greatness: "thick and unpenetratable."

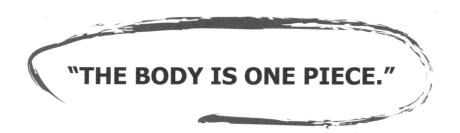

"THE BODY IS ONE PIECE."

Your lats, the "super muscles," as we call them at StrongFirst for their vital contribution to strength and shoulder and back safety, will go live and learn how to play with the other kids. Your shoulder stabilizers will get freakishly strong.

"Stabilizers are what give you the mechanical advantage to be stronger," explains Gray Cook. "This is how the get-up makes you stronger."

Many a bench presser has scratched his head seeing his press climb after getting serious about the get-up. Although the S&S program does not have a pressing exercise in the literal sense, expect your pressing strength to go up. This is in part due to the hypertrophy of the muscles of the shoulder girdle. Science and experience teach us that prolonged isometric contractions build muscle.

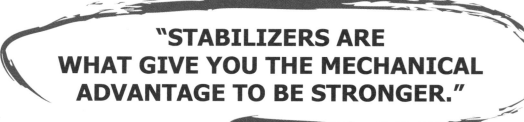

"STABILIZERS ARE WHAT GIVE YOU THE MECHANICAL ADVANTAGE TO BE STRONGER."

The Get-Up Drills

Let us drill your get-up in stages. Follow Karen Smith, Master SFG.

To Elbow

You are about to do a right-handed get-up. Lie on your back with your left arm on the ground, pointing towards your feet at a 45-degree angle. Place your left leg parallel to the left arm.

Straighten your right arm, and place a sneaker (a smelly one, preferably, to better motivate you not to drop it) on top of your upright fist. This odd tactic will enable you to understand the movement without worrying about the weight. The shoe falling off means you have either failed to keep your arm vertical (the only way to go with a heavy weight), or you have made a jerky transition, which is also a no-no.

Bend your right knee and plant the right foot away from your left thigh, pointing the foot approximately 45 degrees to the right. Do not place the heel too close to the glute.

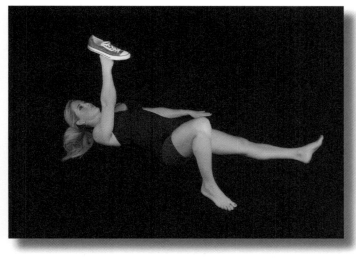

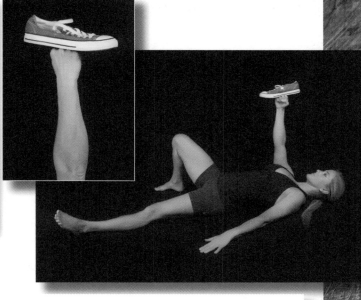

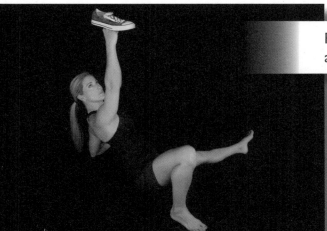

Pushing off your right foot, pivot on the left elbow, and prop yourself up on that elbow.

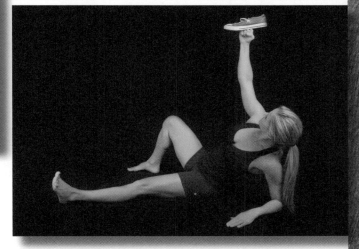

Throughout the evolutions, keep your right wrist rigid; do not extend it to cheat to make supporting the shoe easier. Keep that elbow straight at all times.

This movement is not a crunch or a sit-up. "As you are driving with the planted foot, imagine you are trying to send your chest toward the unloaded side," instructs Mark Toomey, Senior SFG. "Lead with the chest, not with the head. This will prevent neck flexion and strain and create space in the shoulder."

Push your chest out, and your shoulders down away from the ears.

This get-up stage is a remarkable abdominal exercise once you load it.

Practice in sets of five reps until you can do this in your sleep. Precisely control the movement on the way up and down. Do not hold your breath in the get-up evolutions. This is a Yin exercise.

To Hand

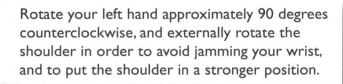

Rotate your left hand approximately 90 degrees counterclockwise, and externally rotate the shoulder in order to avoid jamming your wrist, and to put the shoulder in a stronger position.

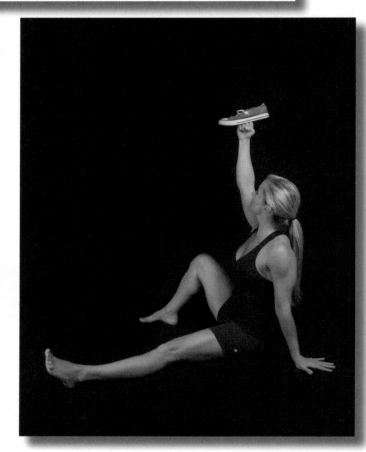

Some people may need to slide the hand back. You will have to experiment to find the your structure's optimal hand placement. It helps to conduct a mental experiment: "If I had to support 100 pounds overhead, where would I want my hand to be?"

Reload the palm while straightening the elbow, pushing your chest out and anti-shrugging the shoulder down. Turn your elbow pit forward as much as possible, without turning the palm.

Push your right knee, which up until now has been pointing inward, out to direct the leg drive. This makes space to sit up. Lengthen your spine to a "tall sit" position.

Turn your head a few times. Turning your head at this and other stages of the get-up helps assure the neck is relaxed and the shoulders are down.

Slowly reverse the sequence, carefully tucking your elbow to the floor.

Remember, look at the kettlebell for the duration of this phase.

To Lunge

There are several ways to progress to the next position, the bottom of the lunge. In this drill you are going to use a "low sweep."

Bend your left knee and tuck the heel in as if you are about to sit cross-legged. Push down hard with your left palm and lift your pelvis to allow the left leg to be swept to the right until the knee is in a line between the right heel and the left hand. You will end up in a windmill position with the right hip hinged to the side, the spine rotated but not bent in any direction.

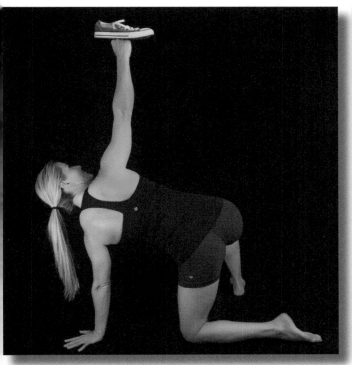

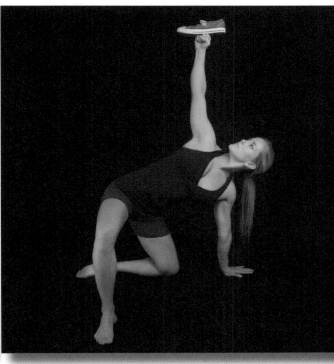

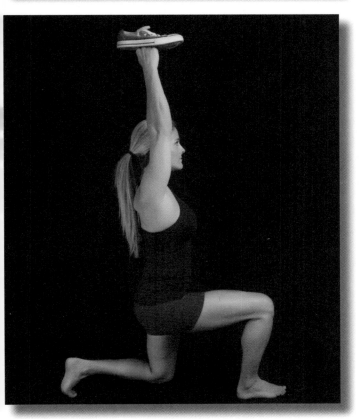

Simultaneously straighten your body upright and square your hips. Tensing the right glute helps.

You are now in the bottom of the lunge position, with your left knee facing left. Square off your hips so the left knee points forward, flex your left foot and place your toes and the ball of the foot on the deck, ready to lunge.

At this point fix your gaze forward toward the horizon and do not look up until you have reached the same point on the way down. You will no longer be looking at the bell.

As with all stages, drill this until it becomes second nature before moving to the next step.

The Tactical Get-Up

Gun-carrying professionals need to be able to quickly assume a kneeling position without losing an upright posture and with minimal use of the hands. For them a roll-up is a better way than a low sweep to reach the half-kneeling position.

Once you have positioned your feet as in the low sweep, push back with the left palm, simultaneously tense both of your glutes and drive the hips forward as you would in a swing. Do not lead with the shoulders.

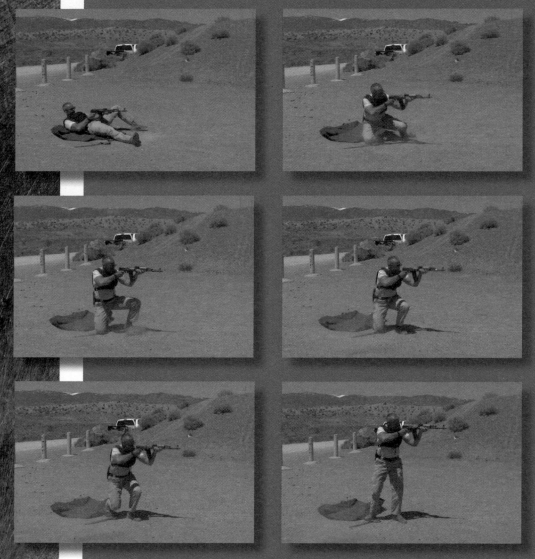

Mark Toomey, Senior SFG performing a tactical get-up with an AKM and an 80-pound vest.

Practice the roll-up without a weight and without your arm raised. Eventually you'll progress to roll-ups without using the planted hand at all.

While it does not challenge the shoulder in as many planes as the low sweep, the roll-up demands greater upper back mobility to keep the raised arm vertical.

Stand Up

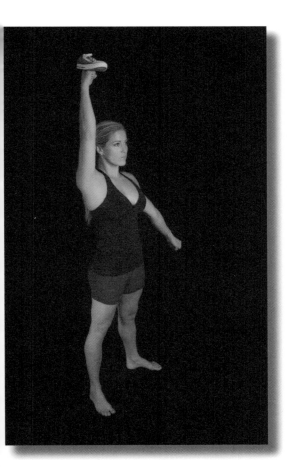

Do not plant your right foot too close to your butt; this would force your knee too far forward on the ascent to the standing position. Experiment to find the sweet spot. Make sure to keep your heel down for the sake of your knee.

Bring your right arm back so it is in line with your ear. Grunt, fire the right glute, and stand up.

Visualize squeezing your knees together when standing up. This will give you a lot more control. Gun-carrying professionals, take a note of this technique for moving from a low shooting position.

You will need to experiment to find a comfortable lunge length and width.

Get Down

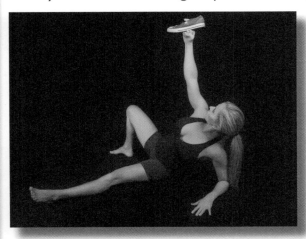

Next you will reverse the get-up from standing to lying.

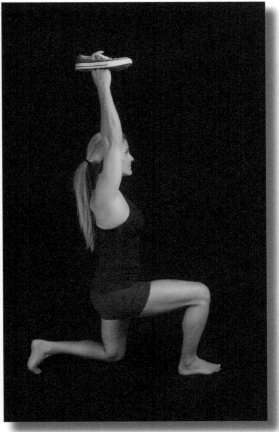

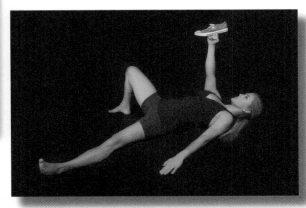

Helpful pointers:

- Step back with your left foot while keeping your weight on the right. Slide your left foot straight back, as if on skis rather than tight-roping it behind the right.

- Touch the deck softly with your left knee. Practice hitting the sweet spot.

- Pivot your left knee so it is facing left—the same position it ended up in after the low sweep.

- Place your left hand on the ground, in line with your left knee. Make sure not to plant the left hand very far from your torso as this would make your left shoulder vulnerable, and could hyperextend your back. Focus not on reaching the ground with your hand, but on hinging the hips sideways to the right.

- Load your lat from the armpit when planting your left hand on the ground.

- Watch out for flexing the right elbow on the way down. Visualize "pushing yourself away from the kettlebell."

- Don't hit the ground hard—you could end up with a kettlebell stuck in your grill.

- If you are too tired or venturing into a new weight territory, you may skip the get-down. Lower the kettlebell to your chest with both hands, then swing it back between your legs, both hands on the handle in a pistol grip, and park it in front of you as you do after swings. I insist that you do use both hands, even if you feel you do not need to.

If any position does not feel right, pause and tweak it.

"The get-up is a slow exercise and there is never an excuse to be out of position," stresses Brett Jones, Master SFG. Take your time and adjust, with or without a bell in your hand—but especially with a bell.

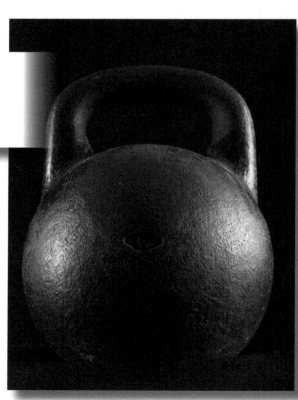

To check your technique at every stage of the get-up ask yourself, "Would I be willing or able to do this with a 100-pound kettlebell?"

Practice this shoe get-up, drilled in stages and as a whole, until you own the movement.

Then enter the kettlebell.

"WOULD I BE WILLING OR ABLE TO DO THIS WITH A 100-POUND KETTLEBELL?"

Pick Up, Set Down, Switch Sides

Lie on your right side, the kettlebell on the ground next to your ribs. Grip the handle with a two-handed pistol grip—the right holding the handle, the left reinforcing the right with a thumbless grip.

Roll onto your back with the kettlebell held tight against your lower ribs. Press the bell upward with one or both arms.

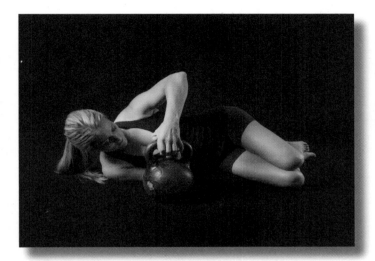 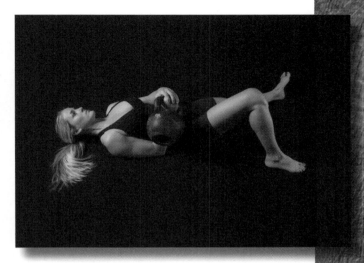

Grip the handle medium hard. Keep the handle parallel to the callus line and wrap your thumb around the handle. Keep your wrist straight—as you would when punching. If you let the wrist bend back, you are telling the world you have never been in a street fight, you big sissy.

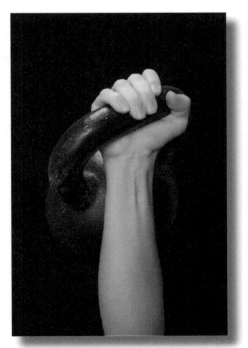 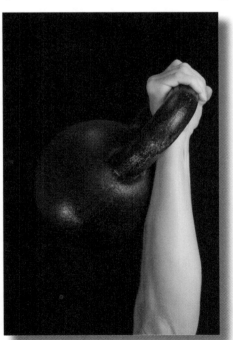 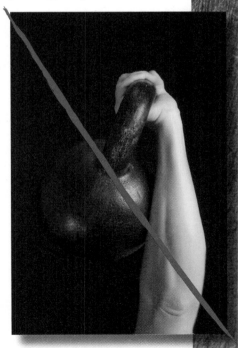

Reverse this process to set the bell back down.

To switch sides perform a lying half-halo, or sit up and spin around. Do not shift the kettlebell over your chest or face.

Look at the bell during the get-up stages unless I tell you otherwise.

Shoulder Packing

The objective of the get-up is not simply standing up with a weight overhead, but doing it while maintaining perfect shoulder mechanics.

Your shoulder is at its strongest and most resilient when it is "packed"—down and sucked into its socket. To learn shoulder packing, raise your right arm overhead, then bend your elbow to reach your mid-back. Restrain your elbow with your left hand try to straighten out your right arm overhead. Note that your shoulder has retreated into your body like a turtle's head.

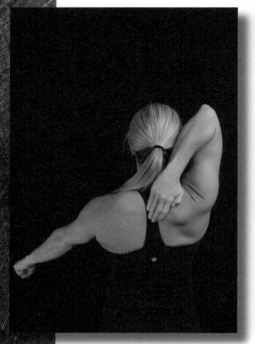 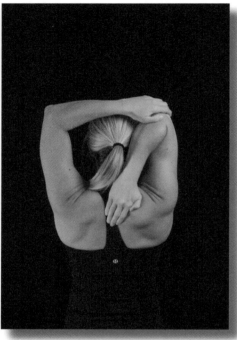 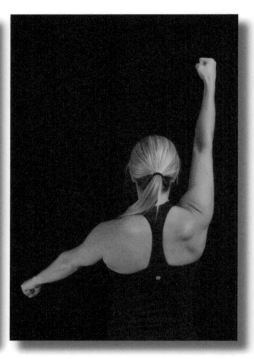

You must keep your elbow straight for the duration of the get-up. This is not for the sake of your elbow, but for the sake of the shoulder—elbow flexion compromises shoulder packing. Visualize a power source in the locked elbow. This sends energy up the forearm into the kettlebell and down into the shoulder. Simultaneously, the arm is "growing longer" toward the kettlebell and pressing hard into the shoulder socket.

It takes effort to keep your elbow straight; do not be lazy.

The left shoulder must be packed too. In this context packed means being pressed down, away from the ears. Revisit the anti-shrug from the short-stop drill in the deadlift section.

Learning to pack your shoulders and building packing strength will make your shoulders bulletproof.

Breathing Behind the Shield

Throughout the get-up, "breathe behind the shield," as they say in some karate styles. Imagine lying on your back with a large person sitting or even standing on your stomach. You would have to brace the abs in order not to get crushed, and then breathe behind that "shield." The breathing would have to be shallow, because deep breaths would collapse the shield.

The *Kata* of The Get-Up

If the swing can be compared to *tameshiwari*—board and brick breaking—the get-up can be thought of as a *kata*, a series of choreographed martial arts movements.

The swing is a Yang exercise; the get-up is a Yin. It stands to reason the speed recommendation for swings is reversed for get-ups—go slow.

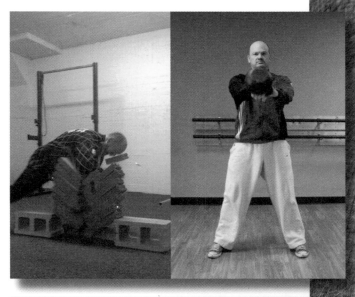

DO SWINGS FASTER THAN COMFORTABLE— GET-UPS SLOWER THAN COMFORTABLE.

Dr. Mark Cheng, Senior SFG, teaches get-ups at a "Tai Chi speed." In Gray Cook's words, if you are unable to do a non-ballistic movement slowly, "you are hiding something."

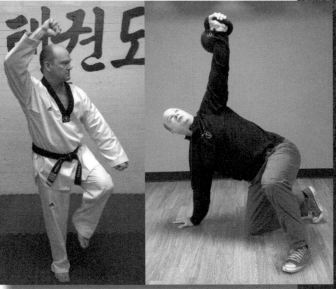

Photos courtesy of Jon Engum

IF YOU ARE UNABLE TO DO A NON-BALLISTIC MOVEMENT SLOWLY, "YOU ARE HIDING SOMETHING."

Pay attention to the insights into kata practice that the accomplished karateka Goran Powell learned from his master.

> One evening [Shihan Chris Rowen] demonstrated a kata both soft and then hard-soft. During the soft kata, he performed each move at a medium pace, with complete relaxation. As he rose onto one leg and prepared to kick, I noticed a small, almost imperceptible wobble. He sunk his weight to steady himself, and for a brief moment, he was completely still. The he let fly with the kick and continued.

When he performed the same kata in a hard-soft style, there was no sign of the wobble. I realized why. By doing the kata slowly first, he was exposing his own slight imperfections in balance and correcting them. He body was learning exactness and correctness. When he sped up, his balance had been recalibrated. It was perfect. It was awesome to watch.

If you always do katas hard and fast, you can hide imperfections with bluster and power. But this is simply papering over the cracks. Doing a kata more slowly, without tension, allows you to dwell on your weaknesses and correct them. Once you speed up again, your movements are much more natural and effective.

This is the mindset for your get-up practice. But just like a martial artist who does kata but does not spar is not a fighter, a person who practices the get-up but does not increase the weight is not a girevik.

"The goal is to have good form, but do not stop there. Own your alignment and lift something," insists Gray Cook.

Get-up Standards

Task:

Get-up

Condition:

Lie on your back, pick up a kettlebell with both hands, and press it with one or both arms. Slowly stand up, proceeding through a low sweep while keeping your loaded arm straight and vertical. Assist yourself by pushing into the ground with the free arm. Slowly reverse the movement from standing to lying.

Standard:

1. Use both hands to lift the kettlebell off the ground to the starting position of the floor press and to return it to the ground at the end of the get-up.

2. The wrist on the kettlebell side is neutral.

3. The elbow on the kettlebell side is locked and the shoulder is packed.

4. The shoulder of the free arm does not shrug up.

5. The heel of the foot on the kettlebell side stays planted during the low sweep, the lunge up to standing, and during the reverse of these actions.

6. The knee touches the deck silently on the descent into the half-kneeling position.

7. The arm holding the kettlebell is vertical or almost vertical.

8. The neck is neutral for the top half of the movement, from the lunge up.

9. In the top position the knees are locked and the lower back does not hyperextend.

The movement is smooth, without jerky transitions.

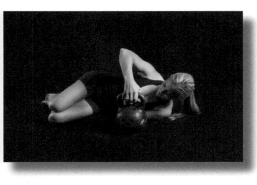
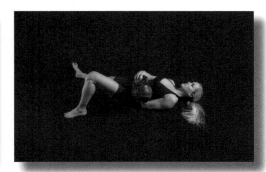

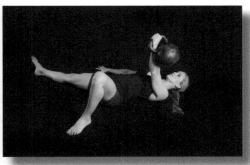

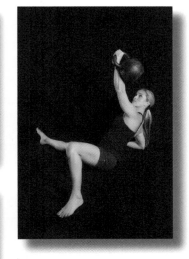

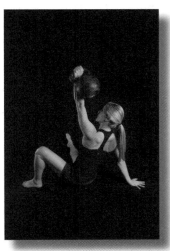

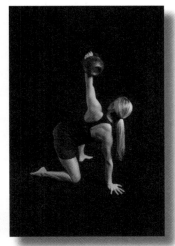

Practice your swings and get-ups, as well as drills leading up to them, for 30 minutes every day after a joint mobility session of goblet squats, SF hip bridges, and haloes. Do not progress to the Program Minimum that follows until your swings and get-ups are competent.

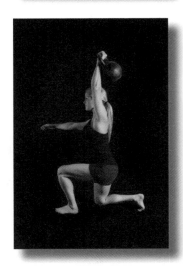

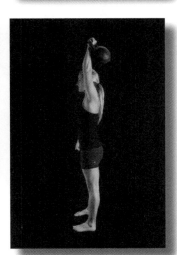

PROGRAM MINIMUM REMASTERED

Get yourself a Glock and lose that nickel-plated sissy pistol.

—Tommy Lee Jones in *U.S. Marshalls*

The Glock pistol has a rare distinction of being the choice of gun-carrying professionals, and the number one pistol recommended to beginners at the same time.

In the 1980s the Austrian armed forces announced a competition for a contract to replace an obsolete WWII-era pistol. Gaston Glock, an engineer with no firearms experience, decided to try his luck. As the story goes, a couple of colonels sniggered that "a man who made curtain rods for a living" did not stand a chance. Herr Glock got mad and went to work. They say he test-fired his prototypes with his left hand. That way if a gun blew up he could still work on blueprints with his right.

This amateur proved the experts wrong. Unburdened by an insider's knowledge of what was possible and impossible, Glock designed a simple and sinister tool that had a lot fewer parts than its competitors. The rest is history. Today Glock is the most popular handgun in the world, supplying two-thirds of the law enforcement agencies in the US and countless institutional and private customers worldwide.

Like the Glock pistol, the Program Minimum (PM) was designed to be a great shooting program, perfect for beginners, the advanced, and anyone in between. Like its second amendment counterpart, the PM was designed by an outsider.

Steve Baccari is a hard man from Boston. An electrician by trade, a fighter by choice, a strength coach by accident. Baccari does not suffer fools or fitness professionals gladly—or at all. He has no tolerance for big words and the only proof he accepts is results.

This man with no formal education understands the scientific method—unlike so many people who flaunt "transverse plane" and "Krebs cycle" jargon. He severely limits the number of variables and tracks one while keeping the rest constant. Two groups of fighters of similar ability are doing the same things—except for one variable—for a certain number of weeks. The proof of what works better comes out in the ring.

I have been to Steve's basement, where I saw a thick stack of notebooks going back a couple of decades. Over the course of his career, he tried everything and ruthlessly eliminated what did not work. From his disciplined and unorthodox mind came the original Program Minimum.

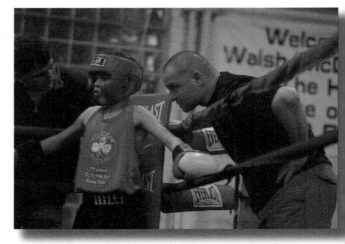

Steve in the corner of young Peter Welch at Saint Patrick's Day Boxing.

Photo courtesy of Steve Baccari

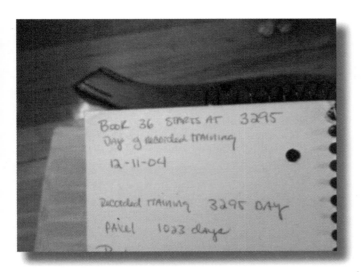

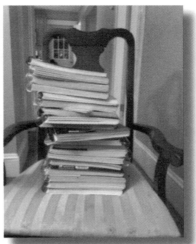

Mad scientist's notes.

Photos courtesy of Steve Baccari

The PM was built with only two parts: the swing and the get-up. Baccari's experience, and later that of many others, has taught us that these two exercises supply the biggest bang for the kettlebell buck.

Like a Glock pistol of an earlier generation, the remastered PM is the same great product, refined.

You will start by training every day, taking an occasional day off when your body insists, or when your schedule puts you in a crunch.

Here is your training session for the first couple of weeks: swings and get-ups.

	Sets times reps	Average strength lady	Strong lady	Average strength gentleman	Strong gentleman
Swings	5x10 (total)	16kg	16kg	24kg	24kg
Get-Ups	5x1 (per arm)	8kg	12kg	16kg	24kg

Train any time of the day. Start with three circuits of mobility exercises—prying goblet squats, hip bridges, haloes.

As an option, you may follow these with a couple of sets of get-ups with exaggerated slowness and precision with a shoe or a light kettlebell. Groove the movement. Instead of doing full get-ups, you may select a particular phase, say supine to elbow, and polish it. Take the movement apart and put it back together. This is not a warm-up, but a practice.

Then do five sets of ten swings, mostly two-arm swings at this stage, occasionally adding a couple of sets of one-arm or hand-to-hand swings. A couple of months down the road when your one-arm swing is solid, it will be the only version you will be using.

When we count swing reps, we add the number of times the kettlebell has swung up and down and pay no attention to what the arms do. For instance, 10T + 10T + 10L + 10R + 10T is 50 swings. "T" stands for two-handed.

On the other hand, when the program tells you to do five get-ups, this means five per arm, which is exactly what you will do after the swings—five sets of one get-up left and five right.

This workout is not a circuit; do all sets of swings before moving on to get-ups.

Ivan Ivanov and other specialists have concluded that ten is the maximum number of reps one can maintain a maximal power output with a submaximal load in a ballistic effort such as the swing.

Get-ups are limited to singles. This is first for safety, as something is bound to give out if you keep a pseudoisometric exercise like the get-up going too long. Second, we do this to prioritize strength development. A single get-up rep on one side lasts about 30 seconds. If you were doing bench presses, you would be able to do about eight clean, paused reps in that time. Sets of eight build strength. Sets of sixteen or twenty-four reps just pump you up.

We do not tolerate weakness at StrongFirst. You do not have a weak arm and a strong arm—but a strong and a stronger one. We owe this discovery to David "Iron Tamer" Whitley, Master SFG.

Start the get-up session with your strong arm. In other words, do a get-up with your left, provided you are right-handed. Lower the kettlebell to the deck with both hands. Pivot your body so the kettlebell is now on your right side. Get up. Do just one rep per arm.

If your get-ups start to get shaky, do partial reps—stop at the stage of the lift where you still feel safe and in control.

Do not rush; "explore the movements," teaches Dan John.

DO NOT RUSH, "EXPLORE THE MOVEMENTS."

Walk around between your sets and shake off tension. Actively rest until your breathing is halfway down to normal.

Rif uses a simple rule of thumb: You are ready for the next set when you can talk again. "This builds an instinctive quality that is important," explains the Master SFG. "The talk test is solid. I don't want to rob the next set of intensity by starting out of breath."

"It is way too easy to lose focus on practice and skill development, not to mention base strength, when you are chasing the clock," warns Reifkind.

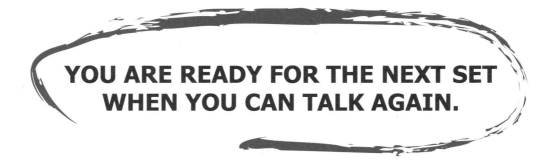

YOU ARE READY FOR THE NEXT SET WHEN YOU CAN TALK AGAIN.

You are to do nothing else during this practice—only lift the kettlebell and move for active recovery. There is no chatting, looking at members of the opposite sex, watching TV, fooling around with your phone (absolutely no phone), taking a drink of water, or going to the bathroom. Just training. Your session is barely half an hour long; stay focused.

> # YOU ARE TO DO NOTHING ELSE DURING THIS PRACTICE—ONLY LIFT THE KETTLEBELL AND MOVE FOR ACTIVE RECOVERY.

These two exercises are very demanding on the grip. Do yourself a favor and help it recover by periodically working the antagonistic muscles between sets. Buy a bundle of broccoli and take off the rubber band holding it together. Throw away the broccoli, then put the band around the fingers and thumb of one hand. Open the fingers against the resistance. No need to push this exercise hard; it is a form of recovery. Do not bother counting reps.

To spare the environment from decomposing broccoli, you may want to buy a set of rubber bands specially made by IronMind.com for finger extensor training.

Stay with the above volume—the total number of reps—until you fully recover from day to day. If you are out of shape, this might take weeks. If you are in great condition, it will take a couple of days.

Then increase the swing volume by 50%, keeping the get-up volume the same.

	Sets times reps
Swings	7-8x10 (total)
Get-Ups	5x1 (per arm)

When you can comfortably get through that workout and the morning after, if your energy is high and soreness is minimal, up the swing total again.

	Sets times reps
Swings	10x10 (total)
Get-Ups	5x1 (per arm)

Meanwhile, read Part II to get a firmer grasp of this program.

Power to you!

PART II: SINISTER

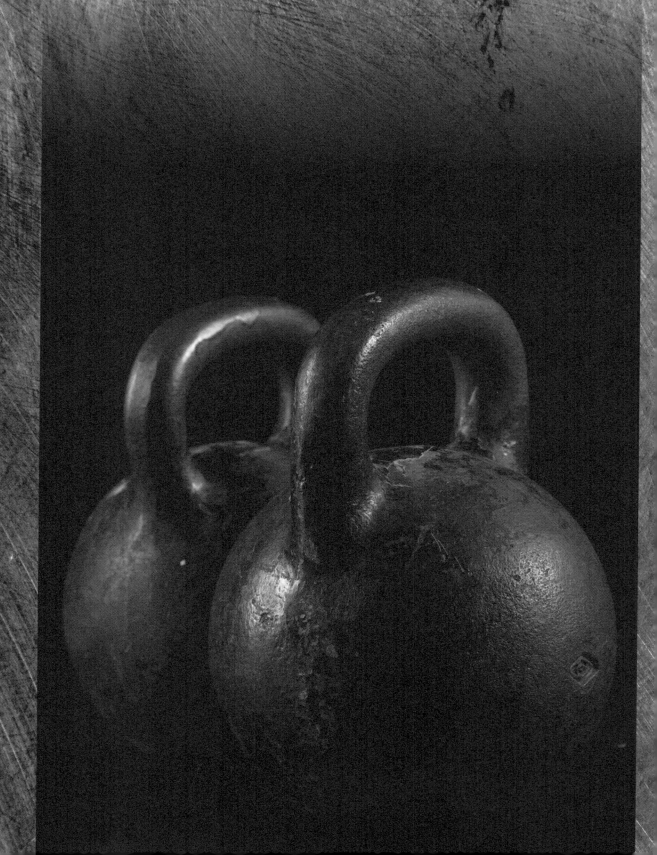

HARD STYLE

When you train, you should train as if on the battlefield. Make your eyes glare, lower your shoulders, and harden your body. If you train with the same intensity and spirit as though you are striking and blocking against an actual opponent, you will naturally develop the same attitude as on a battlefield.

—Ankō Itosu, Okinawan karate master

At StrongFirst we teach the "hard style" of kettlebell training born in the spec ops of the Soviet Union. In the 1970s select units adopted a karate-based style of hand-to-hand combat. The hard style of kettlebell training evolved in the 1980s to support the hard style of fighting.

"WHEN YOU TRAIN, YOU SHOULD TRAIN AS IF ON THE BATTLEFIELD."

In the martial arts context, "hard style" refers to schools that meet force with force and greatly value physical strength.

"The essence of karate techniques is *kime*," explains karate great Masatoshi Nakayama. *Kime* is usually translated as *focus*. "The meaning of kime is an explosive attack to the target using the appropriate technique and maximum power in the shortest time possible." The master reminds us of karate's "one strike, one kill" history to stress the importance of an all-out effort.

"A technique lacking *kime* can never be regarded as true karate, no matter how great the resemblance to karate," continues Nakayama. The karate master stresses that the same is true in non-contact sparring—one must use full force and focus.

StrongFirst has the same attitude. For us "hard style" is the "one strike, one kill" ancient karate philosophy applied to strength training.

"HARD STYLE" IS THE "ONE STRIKE, ONE KILL" ANCIENT KARATE PHILOSOPHY APPLIED TO STRENGTH TRAINING.

Do not hold back. This is hard style.

John "Roper" Saxon, Bruce Lee's co-star in *Enter the Dragon*, told me Bruce Lee showed him the kettlebell swing the day they met. Lee would freeze the kettlebell momentarily on top of each swing to work on focusing the power of his punches. That is kime. This is exactly how we swing at StrongFirst.

"Come up with tremendous power to lock out. Don't play passive." This is how powerlifting world champion Donnie Thompson swings. This is kime. Thompson took his deadlift from 766 to 832, and added 100 pounds to his bench press in nine months with hard style kettlebell training.

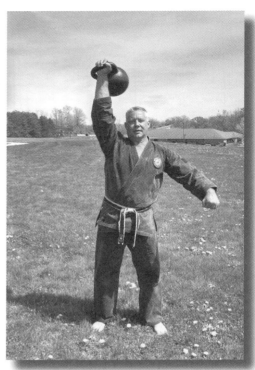

Gary Music, SFG, a 6th degree black belt in Shurite Kempo presses a 48kg "Beast".

Photo courtesy of Gary Music

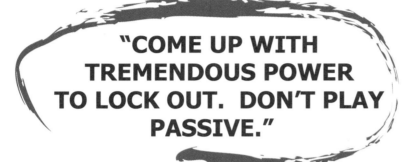

"COME UP WITH TREMENDOUS POWER TO LOCK OUT. DON'T PLAY PASSIVE."

Strength training authority Dr. Fred Hatfield points out that at least 75% of a conventional weight training set is wasted. Only certain parts of the lift are hard, and only the last reps. The rest is just semi-work and momentum. Hatfield instructs pushing as hard as possible against the weight every inch of the way and on every rep.

$F=ma$. Force equals mass multiplied by acceleration. Within reason you can make a given weight as "heavy" as you want by accelerating it. "Now what took a lifter four workouts to accomplish in the gym, takes a lifter using compensatory acceleration only one workout," states Dr. Hatfield, who used compensatory acceleration training (CAT) to achieve one of the first 1,000-pound squats. He trained countless elite powerlifters, football and basketball players, and other athletes with great success.

WITHIN REASON YOU CAN MAKE A GIVEN WEIGHT AS "HEAVY" AS YOU WANT BY ACCELERATING IT.

Hatfield advocates exploding for improving cardiovascular efficiency as well. He specifically recommends explosive rhythmical lifting with relaxed pauses between reps. "Each repetition should be an all-out effort as well—maximum contracture against submaximal resistance, so multiple reps can be performed." Sounds familiar?

Hard style training is also highly effective for fat loss. In a study that compared the energy expenditures in the same exercise performed explosively and non-explosively, the former predictably burned more calories. "The swing is inefficient, which is why it is a great fat burner," explains Dan John. "The bike is efficient—and fat people can ride it forever."

Yes, you could burn the same calories by doing more reps with less power or less weight, but why?

Famous economist Milton Friedman was visiting a construction site in a country with Soviet-influenced economic policies. It was in the 1960s and Friedman was shocked to see only shovels and no mechanized equipment. He asked the government bureaucrat who was giving the tour about it. The latter smugly replied, "You don't understand. This is a jobs program." Prof. Friedman smiled, "Oh, I thought you were trying to build a canal. If it's jobs you want, then you should give these workers spoons, not shovels."

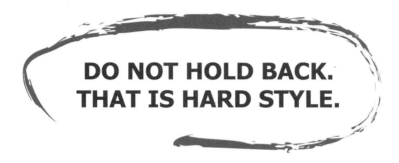

DO NOT HOLD BACK. THAT IS HARD STYLE.

SHADOW SWINGS

> *Jump on a bathroom scale and see what it registers for a split second. The readout is much heavier than your actual bodyweight.*
>
> —Louie Simmons

There is nothing new under the sun. Karate master Nobuyuki Kishi describes "samurai plyometrics" and stresses the value of both concentric and eccentric power training:

> When the samurai wanted to build up the legs and hips, they used to jump over hemp, a plant that grows incredibly fast. Every day the hemp would be higher than before, and the samurai would have to jump higher and higher. This exercise made the legs and ankles strong. This is an example of the "light" element of training. However, when you get older, instead of jumping up over an obstacle, little by little, you can dig a hole and jump into it. This is more of the "shadow" technique.

"Use these two elements," insists the karate sensei—light and shadow, positive and negative. The kettlebell enables us to take shadow training to an entirely new level.

$F=ma$. Force equals mass multiplied by acceleration. One can generate high force by different combinations of "m" and "a."

- High mass and low acceleration—the powerlifts

- Medium mass and medium acceleration—the Olympic lifts and various jumps

- Low mass and high acceleration—the kettlebell swing and various throws

F=MA
FORCE EQUALS MASS MULTIPLIED BY ACCELERATION. ONE CAN GENERATE HIGH FORCE BY DIFFERENT COMBINATIONS OF "M" AND "A."

Soviet sports scientists discovered that a high rate of acceleration on the way down is just as important as on the way up for maximizing athletic performance and resilience. Obviously, you cannot swing a barbell between your legs, and a dumbbell stiffens the shoulders and scares the knees. One solution is depth jumps—jumping off heights as the samurai did. Unfortunately, depth jumps do not spoil you with mass and acceleration choices. Your bodyweight and one "G" is all you get.

Enter the kettlebell. Its shape and compact size allow one to safely accelerate it on the way down in swings and snatches—a so-called overspeed eccentric. Our instructors have been clocked swinging a 24kg bell down with almost 10G, making it "weigh" over 500 pounds.

This is "virtual force," but its effects are very real.

If I set a 24kg kettlebell on your foot, you will find it annoying.

If I drop the same bell on your foot from my chest level, you will need crutches.

If I slam the bell down from the same height, you will need a new leg.

Virtual force need not be destructive. Behold heavier deadlifts, higher jumps, and hamstrings that can take sudden stops and changes of direction.

Even people whose bodies can no longer tolerate static loads of deadlifts and other heavy lifts are able to safely train with very high forces with shadow swings. For many hard men with high mileage, virtual force is the only way to stay in the game.

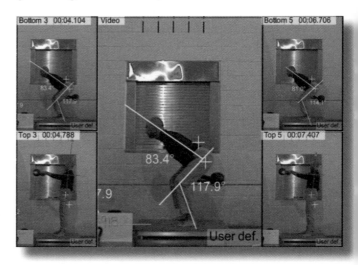

Small caliber, high velocity.

Photo courtesy of Brandon Hetzler

Due to the springiness of our tissues, we can withstand much higher forces if the application is very brief. Imagine getting punched in the ribs by a good boxer with 700 pounds of force. Hospital time. Now imagine lying down and placing 700 pounds of iron on top of your ribcage— on a surface the size of a boxing glove... Cemetary time.

WE CAN WITHSTAND MUCH HIGHER FORCES IF THE APPLICATION IS VERY BRIEF.

Employ overspeed eccentrics or shadow swings only with light kettlebells—30% of your bodyweight or less—and only in two-arm swings. Hike the bell back with all-out acceleration and aggression.

Hard style!

SPEED ENDURANCE IS THE ANSWER

The goal is maximal hip drive, speed and aggression.

—Andy Bolton, the world's strongest deadlifter, on kettlebell swings

Do not allow the kettlebell to slow down during swings—even if the goal is conditioning. The least productive, most exhausting and injury-producing form of resistance training is a high-rep semi-grind—think of the last reps of a long set of pushups or bodyweight squats. Cuban coach Alfonso Duran used to tell young weightlifter Geoff Neupert to stop his sets before his reps slowed down. Today this Master SFG admits that the times he got hurt or overtrained were from not listening to this advice.

HIGH-REP SEMI-GRINDS ARE DANGEROUS, AND ARE NOT PRODUCTIVE.

There are three main muscle fiber types: I, IIA, and IIX.

Type I fibers are slow twitch—small, slow, and weak. They can go on forever, though. It is the marathoner's fiber.

Type IIX are huge and powerful—but they get worn out after a couple of reps. It is the discus thrower's fiber.

The intermediate type IIA is where the money is when you have to produce high forces and maintain them for some time. It is the fighter's fiber.

The S&S swing protocol focuses on the fighter's fiber.

When your reps slow down, it is the best indicator your IIA fast fibers have had it, and slow type I fibers are doing most of the work. This is bad new for several reasons.

First, you are no longer improving your power endurance. Prof. Nikolay Ozolin defined endurance as "the ability to perform work at the desired intensity level for an extended period of time, the ability to fight fatigue and to effectively recover during and after work."

I shall underline the part so frequently missed: *at the desired intensity level*. It does not matter if you can do 1,000 punches if none of them can knock out your little sister.

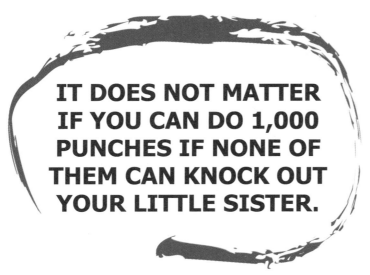

IT DOES NOT MATTER IF YOU CAN DO 1,000 PUNCHES IF NONE OF THEM CAN KNOCK OUT YOUR LITTLE SISTER.

Second, you are more exposed to injury. Chad Waterbury, who has been on the cutting edge of ballistic conditioning for years, offers a great analogy: "Imagine your truck is stuck in the ditch and you have ten guys at your disposal who can pull it out. If you let just three guys pull, it is more likely one of them will get injured because they have to work considerably harder than if all ten guys were pulling on the rope. This is how you should think of motor unit recruitment. There is no reason to do slow-grind reps that overload fewer motor units when you could recruit all the motor units and minimize muscle strain."

Third, once your slow fibers have been pounded, they easily go into spasm, exposing you to injury, compromising your training and the quality of your life. Interestingly, muscles with a high ratio of slow fibers tend to congregate deeper, next to the bones. And slower fibers within any muscle tend to be deeper in the muscle. These two pieces of trivia should give you a hint as to why it is so hard to relieve some knots with massage and foam rollers—they are hard to reach. Do not create the problem in the first place.

These three reasons should be enough to convince you to exercise discipline and stop when your swings are about to slow down—not when something gives out. It may feel like quitting, but it is not. Incidentally, you may use your will power to maintain a high power output rather than to just keep going.

It is equally important that you not only maintain high speed, but finish each rep with a powerful glute cramp and abdominal brace. In addition to building power for knockout strikes and winning deadlifts, this exaggerated glute contraction protects the hip joints and spine. If you can no longer pinch your cheeks, the gig is up. Ditto for your abbies. Failing to tense them at the top of the swing not only robs your power, but endangers your spine.

Watch your breathing, too. If you are no longer able to maintain the hard style breathing rhythm—in on the way down, out on the way up—or if your breathing becomes irregular, the set is over.

STOP YOUR SWING SET BEFORE—

- **YOU SLOW DOWN.**

- **YOU FAIL TO FINISH EACH REP WITH A POWERFUL GLUTE CRAMP AND ABDOMINAL BRACE.**

- **YOUR BREATHING BECOMES IRREGULAR.**

Chad points out that stopping your sets when you are about to slow down will enable you to maintain a very high power output for a long time.

I remember watching a World's Strongest Man competition on ESPN and seeing Mark Felix compete in the "deadlift for reps" event. He was the favorite, but he came in second. Bill "Kaz" Kazmaier interviewed Mark afterward and asked him what went wrong. Mark's response: "I should've rested sooner. Had I done that, I would've gotten two or three more reps."

That's a very telling statement. Speed endurance reps should activate the largest possible range of motor units. Once that range decreases—meaning the speed decreases—the set should be terminated, even if only for a ten-second rest. You would be surprised at the total number of speed reps a fit person could knock out if he rested for just ten seconds as the speed slows down.

"YOU'D BE SURPRISED AT THE TOTAL NUMBER OF SPEED REPS YOU COULD KNOCK OUT IF YOU RESTED FOR JUST 10 SECONDS ONCE THE SPEED SLOWS DOWN."

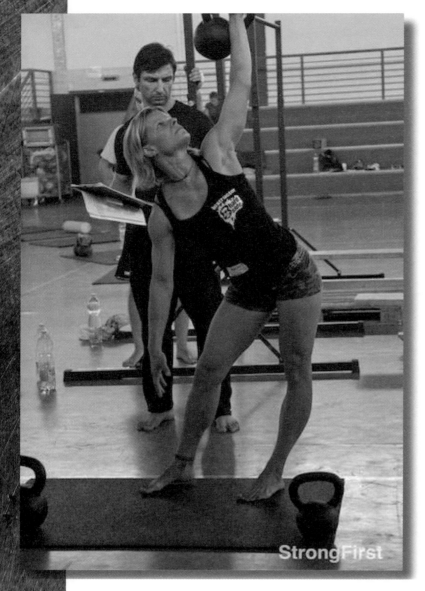

StrongFirst

Rachel "Wolf" Darvas, SFG II, the graphic designer of this book.

Photo courtesy of Peter Lakatos, Master SFG

Dan John has a terrific insight: "Get an idea of when you slow down and train to push the "slow down" rep point higher and higher."

"GET AN IDEA OF WHEN YOU SLOW DOWN AND TRAIN TO PUSH THE "SLOW DOWN" REP POINT HIGHER AND HIGHER."

THE SECRET OF HARD STYLE LAZINESS

Throwing a good punch works like firing a gun. Once the explosion has taken place in the barrel, the bullet flies on its own accord. It accelerates naturally. It does not need to be pushed along.

—Goran Powell, *Waking Dragons*

Do not confuse speed and power with effort.

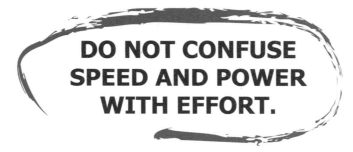

DO NOT CONFUSE SPEED AND POWER WITH EFFORT.

Ballistic events are funny: you will never be at your best when you are trying your hardest.

Explains Prof. Nikolay Ozolin:

> In perfecting the athlete's ability to subjectively evaluate his actions comparison of his sensations during the performance of an exercise in two modes, maximal and near-maximal help the athlete well. This creates a contrast in sensations and subjective evaluations. For instance, a sprinter is instructed to run 30m loosely, without tension, but with an 85-90% effort. He is not told his time. Then the task is repeated, this time with the instruction to run all out, with maximal speed. Afterwards the athlete is told his results and, as a rule, the first number is better.

IN BALLISTIC EVENTS YOU WILL NEVER BE AT YOUR MOST POWERFUL WHEN YOU ARE TRYING YOUR HARDEST.

When I train tactical teams, I teach them the "percentage drill." One guy holds a shield and the other strikes—a punch, a kick, any technique he is skilled at. I tell him to hit as hard as possible several times and instruct the training partner to note the power of each strike. That sets the baseline.

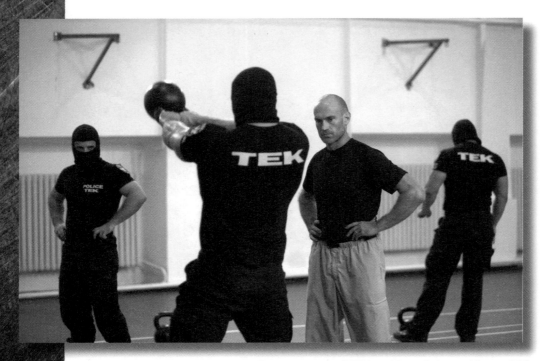

Photo courtesy of TEK and Peter Lakatos, Master SFG

I show the striker a couple of Russian relaxation exercises that look like shaking water off the limbs. Then I explain that I will be ordering him how much effort to put into each strike—50%, 80%, etc. I specify the percentage refers to the effort—not to the speed or the follow-through. Hit as fast as always, follow through the target rather than just tap it.

I take the operator through a dozen or so strikes, going up and down randomly: 50%! 80%! 30%! 90%! 50%! 70%! 80%... I remind him to loosen up between strikes. Then I ask the fellow holding the shield which strikes were the most powerful. Almost universally, experienced fighters hit their hardest at around 80%—and almost as hard at 50%.

ALMOST UNIVERSALLY, EXPERIENCED FIGHTERS HIT THEIR HARDEST AT AROUND 80%—AND ALMOST AS HARD AT 50%.

Brett Jones, Master SFG, explains how to apply this martial skill to the kettlebell swing, using the imagery of a volume knob with settings of one through ten.

> We need to experiment with dialing the volume knob in on the desired settings to find our personal optimal settings. How are we going to do that? During a set of two-armed swings, after a couple of reps, begin to think of a volume or effort setting. Call out in your mind "Number two," and try to hit an effort or volume level of two during that swing. Next rep call out number nine and try to hit that effort or volume level. Next rep hit a four, and then an eight, and then back to a three. Hit all the settings on the volume knob and pay attention to what setting provided the optimal result. Here optimal is defined as a "perfect" swing—crisp and powerful, yet efficient.

You can also vary the "volume" setting from set to set, such as 32kg x 10 @ 50%, 60%, 70%, 80%, 90%, 80%, 50%, 70%, 80%.

Brett continues:

Efficiency is an athletic skill. But efficiency is not soft, or it doesn't have to be. A boxer who throws punches at the optimal level will deliver all the force needed, and be able to go the distance because he can regulate his effort and not wear out by throwing max effort after max effort. Although the max effort is available, it is held in its proper place to be used when needed. Swings are no different. I can dial up a ten or a two, but I still sniff in and brace at the bottom of the swing as I load my hips, and I am still rooting and projecting energy up to a crisp hip finish. This is the essence of balancing tension and relaxation in an athletic sense.

"EFFICIENCY DOES NOT HAVE TO BE SOFT."

Another aspect of going the distance with ballistic lifts is applying force as quickly as possible, and then relaxing. The following passage from the "Karate Way" column in *Black Belt* by Dave Lowry will set you a distant goal to shoot for in your kettlebell swings.

Imagine a video of your reverse punch that's broken down into ten frames. At what point do you begin to tighten the muscles you want to be firm so you make good, solid contact? A new student starts tightening as soon as the movement begins. He is self-conscious about the motion. He is trying to remember technical details. He is using all sorts of energy by squeezing his muscles long before his fist reaches the target. A more advanced practitioner, in contrast, stays loose and relaxed until frame No. 7 or No. 8. At higher levels, the tensing takes place at frame No. 10, the last moment. From there, more mastery comes when you do not tense at the beginning of No. 10 but at the last part of it.

The karateka calls this ability "turning laziness into technical mastery." Note that this kind of "laziness" does not refer to slowing down or weakening the contraction, but to limiting its duration, a very important hard style distinction.

HARD STYLE LAZINESS DOES NOT SLOW DOWN OR WEAKEN THE CONTRACTION, BUT LIMITS ITS DURATION.

Hard style laziness works well only for the strong. Research shows that the stronger the muscle, the less it has to contract to produce a given amount of force. This may sound obvious, but it is profound. Fifty percent of very strong is strong. Fifty percent of weak is irrelevant.

When you own your breath, nobody can steal your peace.

—Anonymous

The ability to fight fatigue and to effectively recover during and after work is a key component of Ozolin's definition of endurance.

RAPID RECOVERY DURING AND AFTER WORK IS A KEY COMPONENT OF ENDURANCE. CONTROLLING YOUR BREATHING DURING REST PERIODS IS ESSENTIAL.

Controlling your breathing during rest periods is essential. Here is a simple exercise practiced in every gym class in the U.S.S.R. that will help you quickly normalize your breathing after a hard set—while benefitting your spine.

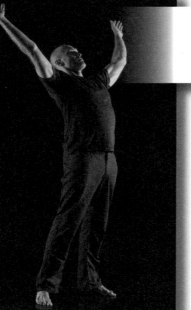

Take a big inhalation, opening your chest and raising your arms overhead in a "Y" shape. Look up, tense your glutes, and slightly bend backward.

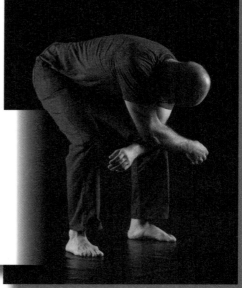

Hold your breath momentarily, then drop your arms and body as if your muscles were suddenly unplugged. Push your tail back and collapse in a hip-hinge pattern, your weight towards your heels. Release a sigh of relief.

Pause for an instant at the bottom, your lungs empty, then stand tall again on a big inhalation.

The above tactic works like a dream when you are sucking wind. However, helping yourself breathe with your arms and body is a luxury you cannot always afford. You need to learn how to calm your breathing without extra movement.

Between bouts of heavy exertion, karate practitioners stand around with deadpan faces and perform *shinkokyuu*—deep abdominal breathing. Rob Lawrence, a senior instructor at my kettlebell school, took this practice a step further. He explains:

> In karate they often told us to breathe calmly, but they did not show us any way of cultivating the skill. The breath-timing technique is designed to do exactly that—teach controlled breathing as a skill.

> The idea is to do a set, take a number of breaths based on some ratio to the number reps you just did, then do the next set. As you will rapidly discover, the way to survive is to slow your breath down as much as possible, to get maximum air and to increase your rest period between each set. If you panic and breathe quickly, your rest period is decreased and you are soon dispatched to the dustbin of history. On the other hand, the only timing involved is your breath—and the idea is to 'cheat' as much as possible by drawing out the breaths and increasing the rest periods.

"THE IDEA IS TO 'CHEAT' AS MUCH AS POSSIBLE BY DRAWING OUT THE BREATHS AND INCREASING THE REST PERIODS."

Not only does such breathing allow you to recover physiologically, it also reduces your stress levels. When we teach our kettlebell instructor courses to special operations teams, on the last day of the course the students are required to put another operator, inexperienced in kettlebells, through a practice and then a workout. We never specify what kind of a workout. Yet almost universally Lawrence's breath timing is prescribed. Professional warriors know the importance of controlling stress in combat and immediately recognize the value of the technique.

The rep-to-breath ratio will vary depending on the exercise and on conditioning. The 2:1 ratio is reasonable for a healthy girevik swinging a moderate-size kettlebell. In other words, ten swings, five breaths.

I strongly urge you to implement breath timing into your daily S&S regimen. It will teach you to breathe properly—through the nose and into the stomach—and under pressure, when you would rather open your mouth and gulp air into your upper chest.

Another breathing technique I am about to teach you will help develop your diaphragmatic breathing, which will help during recovery and in the middle of the swing sets.

Straw breathing is practiced in Russian special operations dive schools to teach economical use of air in the tank, as well as to improve free-diving breath-holding time. As you will see, it can teach you a lot more.

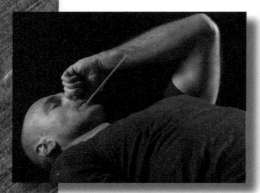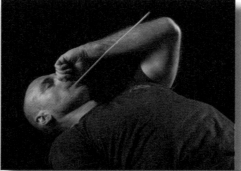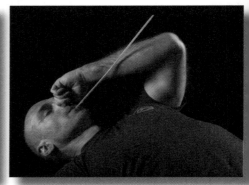

You need several drinking straws. Insert the end of one straw into another about an inch deep to make a long straw. Make a triple straw in the same manner. If the straws get almost plugged up when inserted into one another, tape them together with scotch tape instead of inserting one into another.

Lie on your back with a single straw in your mouth. Pinch off your nose with your fingers, or use a diver's nose clip. Relax, close your eyes, and breathe. That is it. The exercise is what Gray Cook calls "self-correcting."

After a few minutes, replace the straw with two straws. In the beginning you will feel like you are not getting enough air. If you do not panic, you will soon figure out how to adjust your breathing: longer, slower, deeper.

When breathing with two straws becomes comfortable, replace the two with the three. This will notch up the challenge. You will be forced to completely fill and empty your lungs in a very patient manner.

There is no need to add more straws. Have you seen old comic books with a hero walking on the bottom of a river, breathing through a six-foot snorkel? That is impossible, because at a certain length he would be forced to rebreathe the same air trapped in the pipe.

The exercise develops surreal calm. Practice it as often as possible, ten minutes at a shot. Remember its lessons when resting between sets of swings.

In addition, apply one of the lessons to the swing proper. To emphasize the importance of breathing very low into the stomach, karate legend Mas Oyama used the expression "breathing into the groin." To most people this makes no sense. To you, once you have been straw breathing, it will make perfect sense.

During swings you have no business trying to fill your lungs as full of air as you do during recovery breathing. But the "breathing into the groin" cue applies 100%.

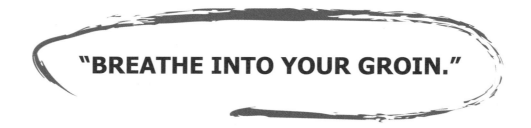

"BREATHE INTO YOUR GROIN."

ANDROID WORK CAPACITY

And suddenly the Hindu Kush was easy.

—Michael Yilek, U.S. Army scout sniper, shortly after starting hard style kettlebell training

In his classic book *Power*, Dr. Fred Hatfield describes an imaginary contest between a 154-pound marathon runner and a 210-pound bodybuilder. Given Dr. Squat's background, it is safe to assume the bodybuilder is not a pump artist, but a power bodybuilder who trains according to Hatfield's recommendations, such as 5x5 squats.

The challenge is carrying twenty 100-pound beer kegs to the pub's second floor as fast as possible. "That's a real feat of endurance, if ever there was one," exclaims Hatfield. Huffing and puffing and not particularly happy, the bodybuilder wins hands down.

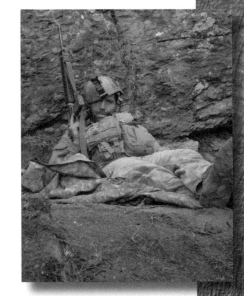

Michael Yilek down range.

Photo courtesy of Michael Yilek

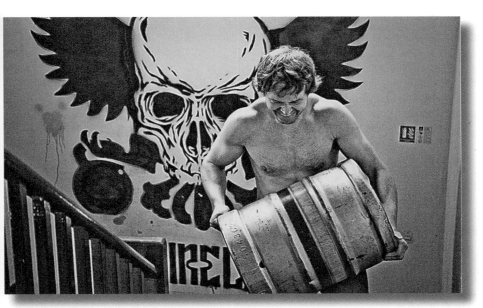

My money is on crazy Irishman Pol McIlroy, SFG II who deadlifts 3.25 times his bodyweight.

Photo courtesy of Pol McIlroy

The second event is carrying 50% of his bodyweight up the same stairs, for time. "It'd be a tossup, I reckon," comments Hatfield, "depending on who was the most motivated by the prize. Even there, I'd put my beer money on the bodybuilder."

Dr. Squat continues his mental experiment. "Try to picture what would happen if the marathon runner had to wear a lead-filled vest to bring his bodyweight up to that of the bodybuilder. Who would win the marathon then? Hell, who'd even finish?"

The sports scientist sums up, "You can devise all sorts of devilish means of proving your own point, depending on who you'd like to see win. The point is, you're still comparing apples and oranges."

Dr. Squat's "apples and oranges" comment refers to endurance specificity. Indeed, there are many types of endurance and dozens of mechanisms responsible for expressing it, from will power to a max VO_2 uptake. If you are serious about a sport, at the point when you are almost a contender, you will need to work with a coach on developing your sport-specific endurance. Otherwise, a reliable general endurance program such as Simple & Sinister is all you need.

In Russian sports science and coaching practice, endurance is subdivided into general and special, meaning sport-specific. "General endurance is the ability to perform for an extended period of time any work involving many muscle groups and placing high demands on the cardiovascular, respiratory, and central nervous systems," explains Prof. Nikolay Ozolin, one of the giants of Soviet sports science. "General endurance is the basis for development of special endurance, which is confirmed by sport experience and research."

"GENERAL ENDURANCE IS THE BASIS FOR DEVELOPMENT OF SPECIAL ENDURANCE."

Note that developing special endurance is the job of your sport coach, your team leader, or your sensei. Mine is to give you a simple and sinister foundation of general endurance for that specialized work.

There are many ways to develop general endurance. In my experience, kettlebell quick lifts are second to none and are the most efficient. When Russians talk about general development, they imply a wide carryover to a great many applications: "...the ability... to perform any physical work more or less successfully." (Ozolin)

Time and time again, kettlebell ballistics have been shown to improve stamina in a great variety of contexts, from running a marathon to fighting full contact to surviving a twelve-hour powerlifting meet.

GENERAL ENDURANCE IS THE ABILITY TO ENDURE "ANY PHYSICAL WORK MORE OR LESS SUCCESSFULLY."

Hard style kettlebell training is highly foolproof. Americans are notoriously poor at following instructions, and yet the Russian kettlebell delivers without fail. Like an AK-47, it tolerates any abuse and keeps doing its job.

Over the years I have received thousands of testimonials concerning the kettlebell's "what the hell effect" on various types of endurance. The routines these folks did were all over the board. Some followed programs written by me or my colleagues, others "improved" them, most cooked up some weird plans of their own that made very little sense to me. They ranged from beginners to elite athletes, and came from a variety of sports and backgrounds. All of them improved, and most of them dramatically.

THERE ARE MANY WAYS TO DEVELOP GENERAL ENDURANCE. KETTLEBELL QUICK LIFTS ARE SECOND TO NONE AND ARE THE MOST EFFICIENT.

If You Like to Argue

It is very tempting for a certain type of a person to nitpick that a given regimen does not give enough attention to the lactate threshold, VO_2 max, or some other valid marker of endurance. I will send him to *Antifragile* by Nassim Nicholas Taleb:

> We are built to be dupes for theories. But theories come and go; experience stays. Explanations change all the time, and have changed all the time in history (because of causal opacity, invisibility of causes) with people involved in the incremental development of ideas thinking they always had a definitive theory; experience remains constant.

> ...Take for instance, the following statement, entirely evidence-based: *if you build muscle, you can eat more without getting more fat deposits in your belly* and can gorge on lamb chops without having to buy a new belt. Now in the past the theory to rationalize was "Your metabolism is higher because muscles burn calories." Currently I tend to hear "You become more insulin-sensitive and store less fat." Insulin, shminsulin; metabolism, shmetabolism; another theory will emerge in the future and some other substance will come about, but the exact same effect will continue to prevail.

> The same holds for the statement *Lifting weights increases your muscle mass*. In the past they used to say that weight lifting caused the "micro-tearing of the muscles," with subsequent healing and increase in size. Today some people discuss hormonal signaling or genetic mechanisms, tomorrow they will discuss something else. But the effect has held forever and will continue to do so.

> I just want to understand as little as possible to be able to look at regularities of experience.

Applied to endurance training, we have known for a long time that heavy swings—and not that many of them—build "conditioning" (whatever it is) extremely well. It did not make any sense, but we rolled with it. May I suggest that you do, too. "A paradox is not a conflict with reality," quipped Richard Feynman. "It is a conflict between reality and your feelings of what reality should be like."

We still know very little about the nature of fatigue—and most of it is supposedly in the nervous system, anyway. In response to max VO_2 uptake and similar arguments in favor of the marathoner, Hatfield cut: "But no one has ever looked at the problem in what I consider to be the right light. By George, the bodybuilder *still* carted those beer kegs up the stairs faster than the runner!"

A LESSON FROM WORKERS AND PEASANTS

Muscles are given to a man not for admiration but for work.

—Prof. Arkady Vorobyev and Yuri Sorokin

Steve Justa is what Marty Gallagher calls an "agro-American." A self-taught strongman from a Nebraska farm. His book *Rock, Iron, Steel*, published by IronMind, is a fascinating insight into what a smart man unburdened by formal education can come up with. I am not going to go on a limb and agree with everything Justa recommends, but I can make a general statement that if one wants to get strong, it is a far better source than most snooty volumes by Ph.D.s with soft hands.

Justa, a muscular 250-pounder with ten years of lifting experience, was taught a lesson when he worked at a foundry. One day he had to take over the station of a worker who had gotten sick, a scrawny 140-pounder. The job entailed clearing warm steel blocks weighing up to 300 pounds from sticky sand by hammering them, picking them up, shaking and dropping them…for the entire shift. Justa recalls, "After a couple of hours of this I was a wreck, physically and mentally, and I kept seeing a picture in my mind of the guy who usually did this job. He was skinny as a rail and he never even worked up a sweat when he was doing this job…"

That day Steve Justa committed to work on his stamina. But what he had in mind was very different from a puke circuit or a high-rep burnout. He decided to do many low-rep sets with a moderately heavy weight, "not to the point of huffing and puffing, but to the point where I could do the movement over and over again for three to five hours if called upon. Of course, take adequate rest between sets, but not so very much rest, and use sets where you're just *slightly tired* at the end of them."

"…NOT TO THE POINT OF HUFFING AND PUFFING, BUT TO THE POINT WHERE YOU CAN DO THE MOVEMENT OVER AND OVER AGAIN."

I am not going to try to convince you to do swings for five hours. I do want you to take note of the working man's attitude to training: "…to the point where you can do the movement over and over again. This is a blue-collar man doing his job. Contrast his mindset with that prevailing among the trainees who fancy themselves hardcore: prey fluttering and desperately trying to save its life.

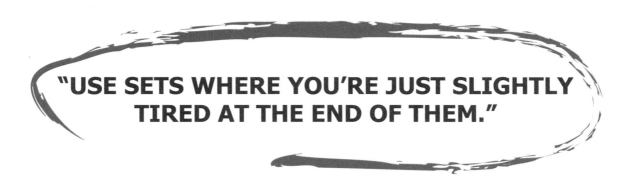

"USE SETS WHERE YOU'RE JUST SLIGHTLY TIRED AT THE END OF THEM."

Like Justa's, my endurance program is heavily biased towards strength, because, as strongman Earle Liederman observed back in 1925, "What is endurance except *continued strength?*"

"WHAT IS ENDURANCE EXCEPT CONTINUED STRENGTH?"

Here is how to apply this frame of mind to swings and get-ups. Think of yourself as a contractor with a job of 100 of one and ten of the other. If it is a job, you naturally want to finish it as quickly as possible, punch out, and go out for beer and pizza. On the other hand, you are not in the mood to kill yourself to the point where you fall asleep with your face in a double pepperoni and extra cheese. And you remember you have another job waiting tomorrow—and the day after, and one after that.

Listen to Rif:

> I come from a gymnastics and powerlifting background, and I like my rest. I prefer to start my next set when my heart rate has come down a bit and I can put my all into the next set… I like intensity as well. It's hard to be intense on the next set when I am still out of breath.

> My way of training the swing is looking at the volume and intensity and not worrying so much about the rest intervals. These will naturally diminish as work capacity and fitness improves, which just lets you handle more weight and go harder. And that ain't easy… Believe me, after a certain point, a longer rest doesn't make things easier—it just drags things out. And, as your condition improves with consistent workouts, your rest periods will naturally come down. I always start off with longer rest periods than I finish with. It takes me a long time to get warmed up, but once I do, I can do a lot of work with little rest.

> And so can you.

> **FOCUS ON INTENSITY—WEIGHT, EXPLOSIVENESS—AND QUALITY, AND DO NOT OBSESS OVER THE REST PERIODS. THEY WILL NATURALLY GET SHORTER.**

No Workers and Peasants' Paradise

Should you get the impression that I am promoting naturalistic training methods such as manual labor, I am not.

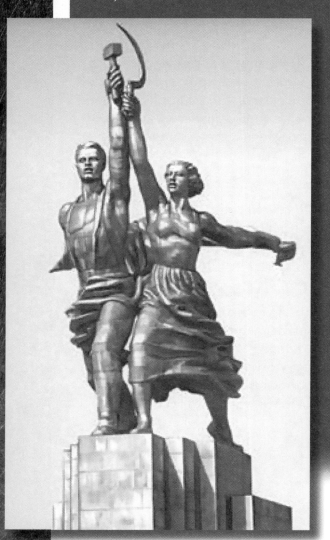

Some forms of it are excellent general exercise. Elite boxing and kickboxing coach Andrey Dolgov used to send his fighters out to the countryside on Boy Scout–type missions. They would knock on old ladies' doors and volunteer to saw and chop firewood.

But more often than not, I would not recommend manual labor as training. Most forms of it develop the body in an asymmetrical manner. Some flat-out cause injuries. Many lack the intensity needed to build real strength.

A few decades ago Soviet scientists brought a bunch of sturdy farm boys to the city with the intention of turning them into weightlifting champions. To the authorities' big disappointment, the collective farmers did not do any better than the city-slickers. Not worse, certainly, just not better.

I am not prescribing a worker's or a peasant's training—only his mindset.

Not the best way to get strong.

A LITTLE EVERY DAY
GOES A LONG WAY

More is not better, it's just more.

—Steve Baccari

Would a higher volume be more effective? Would shorter rest periods?

Perhaps—but at what cost?

"MORE IS NOT BETTER, IT'S JUST MORE."

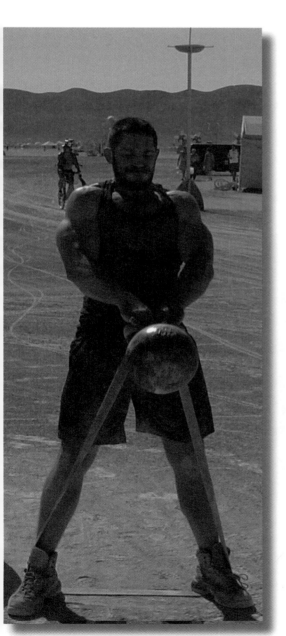

Michael Castrogiovanni, SFG Team Leader.

Photo courtesy of Michael Castrogiovanni

First, consider that StrongFirst puts a premium on strength and power.

It is tempting to write off the kettlebell as only an endurance tool, given its relative lightness. But do not forget the "virtual force" that multiplies the bell's "heaviness" by as much as ten times in the hands of a skilled hard style girevik.

If you are told to do a higher volume or to compress the rest periods, you will unavoidably start holding back power, pacing yourself. Your goal would change from getting the desired training effect to just surviving. Remember Dr. Hatfield's "cardio" training instructions to a power athlete: "an all-out effort… maximum contracture against submaximal resistance."

Another issue is efficiency. Once you reach a certain volume, you hit the point of diminishing returns. The human body is a non-linear system. This means doubling your swings from 100 to 200 will not double the results—far from it. A decade ago Michael Castrogiovanni, today an SFG Team Leader, identified the swing workout that gives the most for the least: 100 swings total, three times a week.

Tim Ferriss, always dedicated to finding the minimum effective dose, discovered that as few as 150-300 weekly swings was the dose for him. A total of ten to twenty minutes of weekly swings got him a ripped six-pack and added over 100 pounds to his deadlift.

100 SWINGS PER WORKOUT IS THE MINIMUM EFFECTIVE DOSE.

Finally, there is the big issue of leaving enough energy for other things—practicing sport skills, being ready to fulfill your duty on the battlefield, or just enjoying your day and not dragging your tail through it.

Bulgarian elite gymnastics coach Ivan Ivanov believes that the purpose of a training session is to store energy in the body rather than exhaust it. That is a powerful mindset. In Ivanov's experience, 100 repetitions per movement hit the spot—and these must be done daily. I concur.

The get-up, due to its semi-static nature and long time under tension, demands much lower sets and reps. Five times one per side look deceptively easy on paper, but hit home once you do them with correct technique and decent weight. Five get-up singles per side keep the muscles under tension for as long as 5x8 benches. This is no walk in the park.

THE PURPOSE OF A TRAINING SESSION IS TO STORE ENERGY IN THE BODY, NOT EXHAUST IT.

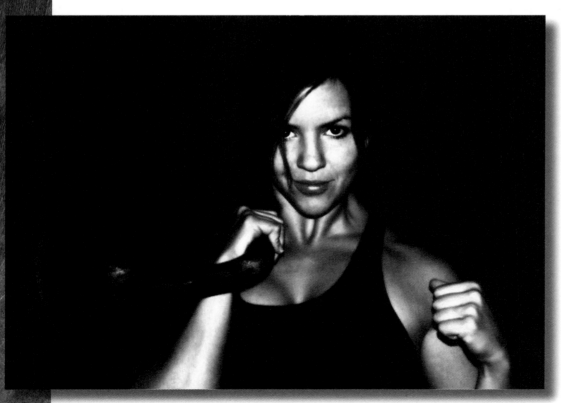

Laura Nepodal, SFG I,
a 325-pound deadlift
with no belt.

Photo courtesy of
Laura Nepodal

It may seem strange to recommend training without days off when the goal is storing energy, but moderate daily training will keep the muscles' fuel tanks topped off, while making tissues resistant to microtrauma and almost soreness-proof. It is the ticket to being always ready.

MODERATE DAILY TRAINING IS THE TICKET TO BEING ALWAYS READY.

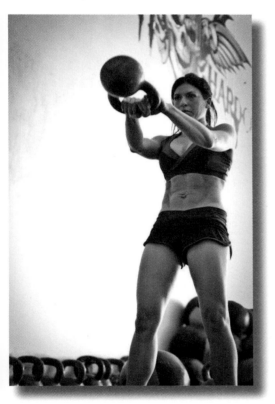

Lauren Brooks, SFG Team Leader can do a strict pullup with a kettlebell that is half her bodyweight on her waist.

Photo courtesy of Lauren Brooks.

Prof. Arkady Vorobyev explains that incomplete restoration training stimulates the recovery ability; your body literally has to learn how to recoup faster…or else. Those who have served in the military can relate. You got sore after your first day in basic training, but you persisted—as if you had a choice—and kept up with the daily grind of pushups and runs, and finally you could handle it. If you were given the unlikely choice of PT-ing only when you had totally recovered, you still would have been stiff, sore, and a sissy. This is why the S&S program, while tolerating a minimum of two workouts a week if you are in a pickle, prescribes near-daily training.

Think of the S&S regimen not as a workout but as a recharge.

One of the meanings of the verb "to work out" is "to exhaust by extraction." Ponder that for a moment and ask yourself if that is your goal. In contrast, "recharge" is the name Russians gave to an invigorating morning exercise session. Out with a workout, in with a recharge!

IT IS NOT A WORKOUT, BUT A RECHARGE.

SIMPLE AS CAN BE

Everything should be made as simple as possible, but not simpler.

—Albert Einstein

I pushed S&S programming to the very edge of Einstein's quote, to the verge of being too simple. I have done this on purpose, in order to eliminate any possible excuse you might have for non-compliance.

The Glock does not have a safety switch. Once the round is chambered, the weapon is ready to fire. Professionals consider this an asset, not a liability. Flipping a tiny safety switch is a fine motor skill. No big deal in the safety of the range, it is a very different matter in a life-threatening situation.

Do you want to be "always ready"? Practice dialing 911 in the dark after a hard set of swings. I am dead serious. In a stressful situation, fine motor skills are compromised. There are many documented cases of people fumbling, unable to call the police. This is why security experts recommend practicing this simple "skill."

Racking the slide and sending the round into the chamber, on the other hand, is a gross motor skill. With practice you can do it quickly with greater reliability than flipping the dainty safety switch. And you will gain a psychological advantage: The clanking of the slide acts like a warning shot to whoever intends to harm you.

For the sake of simplicity, I purposefully removed the equivalent of the safety switch from the S&S program, namely load variability or "waviness," as Russians call it.

Russian coaches learned through trial and error that the higher the volume or intensity, the more "wavy" the programming needs to be. In other words, the harder you push on the heavy days, the easier the light days should be.

The reverse is also true. If you do not have heavy days, you do not need light days.

IF YOU DO NOT HAVE HEAVY DAYS, YOU DO NOT NEED LIGHT DAYS.

Making the training load consistently moderate makes planning training a no-brainer. Just bang out 100 daily swings and ten get-ups like brushing your teeth. All of your attention is on technique and power, and zero brain cells need to be involved in analyzing the workout and planning how to change it.

What an opportunity to become an ultimate technician, just like an old-time strongman! John McKean of the United States All-Round Weightlifting Association explains: "Fixed-poundage sets allowed [old-timers] the security that the lift would always go, so even more attention was devoted to ideal positioning, and perfect angles of push. They never went to the wall (or even wanted to think in terms of any failure) on these sets, where serious breakdown of form could occur, and thus develop bad habits or injury."

Another plus of having a training regimen that does not push limits—you can stay on it for a long, long time. Internet forums rage with the debate of how often one should change a training plan.

It depends.

The more intense the training, the more often the program needs to be changed. For instance, if your deadlift plan is to work up to a max single once a week, it is only sustainable for two to six weeks, with experienced strength athletes on the low end of that range and newbies on the high. This is why lifters who follow the Westside Barbell system that prescribes weekly maxing change the exercises every week or two.

On the other hand, you can stay on Justa's singles routine, which calls for up to fifteen daily singles with a mere 70% of the one-rep max, for as long as you want. I have met gents who casually took their deadlifts from 400 to 500 in a year on this "easy strength" plan.

THE HARDER THE TRAINING, THE MORE OFTEN THE PLAN NEEDS TO BE CHANGED. AND VICE VERSA.

The SFG kettlebell instructor manual describes changing the order of the exercises as an effective means of stimulating continued progress while subtly altering the training effect. For instance, this might mean doing get-ups first, supersetting swings and get-ups, sandwiching the get-ups between 50 swings on the front end and 50 on the back end, and so on.

Nevertheless, I chose not to give you that option in S&S. You have no decisions to make. You are to dedicate 100% of your attention to technique and power.

THE GOALS
AND HOW TO REACH THEM

Swings rock. Heavy swings rock more.

—David "Iron Tamer" Whitley

Stay with whatever weight you are using for a while. Focus on technique in both exercises, and on power in the swing. Gradually reduce the rest periods—but without undue pressure. S&S is an "easy strength" and "easy endurance" program.

Eventually you will reach the point where the work-to-rest ratio is 1:1, which means you will hammer out 100 swings in five minutes and ten get-ups in ten minutes. It is almost time to move up in weight.

Almost.

Rif insists: "When you can do equal work to equal rest on swings and get-ups STRONGLY, not just do it, then move up." This is the attitude of an old-time strongman who refused to move up until he owned his last accomplishment.

Lest you get impatient, I want to remind you that you will still be making progress in strength and conditioning even when you are repeating the same workout over and over. If this were not true, logging and similar jobs would not make men out of boys, and, undeniably, they do.

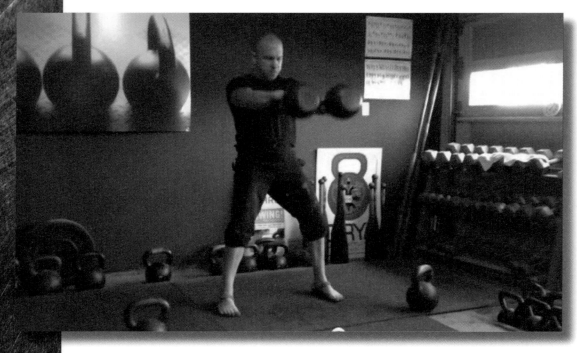

"Rif" in his
"courage corner."

Photo courtesy of
Mark Reifkind

Even though this program is very conservative, life happens and there will be days when your body will tell you to take it easy. Do not turn an off-day into a day off. Easy training is far better than no training.

DO NOT TURN AN OFF-DAY INTO A DAY OFF. EASY TRAINING IS FAR BETTER THAN NO TRAINING.

Cut the weight in both exercises. Make up for it by using "virtual force" in the swings and being extra precise in the get-ups.

The perfect swing weight for an unloading workout is 30% of your bodyweight, which is the sweet spot for power production, according to the research by Brandon Hetzler, SFG Team Leader. Use the two-arm version and employ overspeed eccentrics, the shadow swing.

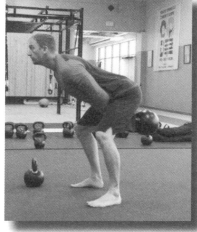

Research by Brandon Hetzler, SFG Team Leader,
helps us keep sharpening our blade.

Photo courtesy of Brandon Hetzler

80

Make your light get-ups evil by adding a ten-second pause at every stage. Ron Farrington, SFG Team Leader, SWAT operator and MMA fighter, promises these pauses will teach you a lot about alignment, breathing behind the shield, fatigue management, and plugging up any leaks preventing your body from becoming one piece.

Light days are not what they are cracked up to be.

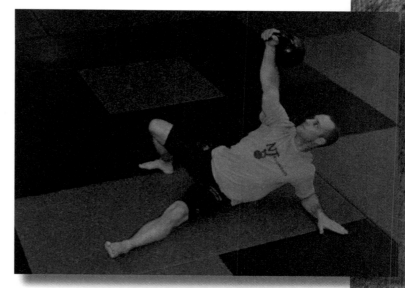

Ron Farrington, SFG Team Leader.

Photo courtesy of Ron Farrington

ON LIGHT DAYS USE TWO-ARM SHADOW SWINGS WITH A KETTLEBELL AROUND 30% OF YOUR BODYWEIGHT OR LESS, AND ADD A 10-SECOND PAUSE AT EACH STAGE OF THE GET-UP.

Back to the progression—do not jump the gun by upping the weight in all the sets. Gradually bump up a set here, a set there.

For instance, a gentleman who owns a 32kg get-up and is ready to take on the 40kg might do the following with each arm.

32, 32, 32, 32, 32	32, 40, 32, 32, 32
32, 40, 32, 32, 32	32, 40, 32, 32, 32
32, 40, 32, 32, 32	—— (day off)
—— (day off)	32, 40, 40, 32, 32
32, 40, 32, 32, 32	32, 40, 40, 32, 32
32, 40, 32, 32, 32	—— (day off)
32, 32, 32, 32, 32 (unloading day)	32, 40, 40, 32, 32
32, 40, 32, 32, 32	32, 40, 40, 32, 32

32, 40, 40, 40, 32	32, 40, 40, 40, 40
32, 40, 40, 40, 32	32, 32, 32, 32, 32 (off day)
32, 32, 32, 32, 32 (unloading day)	32, 40, 40, 40, 40
—— (day off)	32, 40, 40, 40, 40
32, 40, 40, 40, 32	32, 40, 40, 40, 40
32, 40, 40, 40, 32	32, 40, 40, 40, 40
32, 40, 40, 40, 32	—— (day off)
32, 40, 40, 40, 40	32, 40, 40, 40, 40
32, 32, 32, 32, 32 (off day)	32, 40, 40, 40, 40
32, 40, 40, 40, 40	32, 32, 32, 32, 32 (unloading day)
32, 40, 32, 32, 32 (unloading day—realized it was needed after one heavy set)	32, 40, 40, 40, 40
	40, 40, 40, 40, 40

Do not blindly copy the above; it is just an example.

Just learn the lessons:

- Add weight to the second or third set.

- Stay with one heavy set as long as needed to feel ready to add a second.

- There is no specific number of workouts with a given number of heavy sets before adding another. Listen to your body.

- Add no more than one heavy set per training session.

- Do not be afraid to fall back to a lighter weight if you are having an off day, even if you have already started lifting a heavier one.

The following is a sample swing progression for a lady moving up from a 24kg to a 32kg. I am listing the weights for one arm. "24, **32**, **32**, 24, 24" means "24L, 24R, **32L**, **32R**, **32L**, **32R**, 24L, 24R, 24L, 24R."

24, 24, 24, 24, 24	24, 32, 32, 24, 24
24, 32, 24, 24, 24	24, 32, 32, 24, 24
24, 32, 24, 24, 24	20, 20, 20, 20, 20, 20, 20, 20, 20, 20 (two-handed shadow swings—unloading day)
24, 32, 24, 24, 24	
24, 32, 24, 24, 24	24, 32, 32, 32, 24
24, 32, 24, 24, 24	24, 32, 32, 32, 24
—— (day off)	—— (day off)
24, 32, 32, 24, 24	24, 32, 32, 32, 24

24, 32, 32, 32, 24	—— (day off)
24, 32, 32, 32, 24	24, 32, 32, 32, 32
20, 20, 20, 20, 20, 20, 20, 20, 20, 20 (two-handed shadow swings—unloading day)	24, 32, 32, 32, 32
	24, 32, 32, 32, 32
24, 32, 32, 32, 24	20, 20, 20, 20, 20, 20, 20, 20, 20, 20 (two-handed shadow swings—unloading day)
24, 32, 32, 32, 24	
—— (day off)	24, 32, 32, 32, 32
24, 32, 32, 32, 24	24, 32, 32, 32, 32
24, 32, 32, 32, 24	—— (day off)
24, 32, 32, 32, 24	24, 32, 32, 32, 32
24, 32, 32, 32, 24	24, 32, 32, 32, 32
24, 32, 32, 32, 24	24, 32, 32, 32, 32
20, 20, 20, 20, 20, 20, 20, 20, 20, 20 (two-handed shadow swings—unloading day)	32, 32, 32, 32, 32

Again, the above is just an example. You might progress faster or slower.

Once you are doing all the sets with a heavy weight, work on dominating it. Then slowly compress the rest periods. When you are finally able to do 100 swings in five minutes and five plus five get-ups in ten minutes—move up in weight again, using a staggered pattern.

It goes without saying that your swings and get-ups will progress at a different rate. If your swings are at five minutes, you do not need to wait for the get-ups to hit ten before bumping up your swing weight.

I will give you two sets of goals, one simple and the other sinister. The first are easily achievable by most, and you must reach them if you are to enjoy the various benefits of S&S.

SIMPLE GOALS

	Women	Men
100 one-arm swings (sum of arms) in sets of ten in five minutes	24kg	32kg
Five get-ups per arm in sets of one in ten minutes, after the swings and one minute of rest	16kg	32kg

The second set of goals is for an ambitious person determined to earn his man card or her woman card.

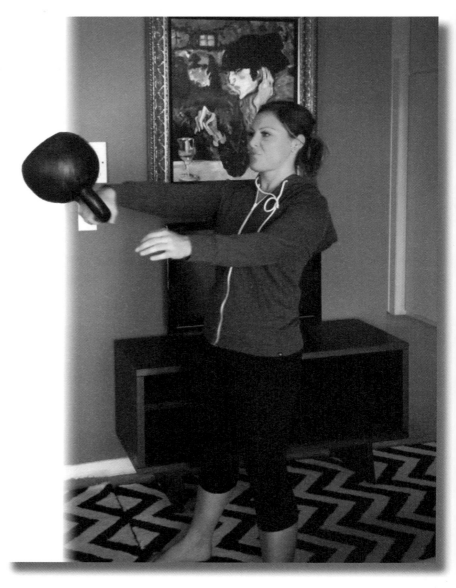

SINISTER GOALS

	Women	Men
100 one-arm swings (sum of arms) in sets of ten in five minutes	32kg	48kg
Five get-ups per arm in sets of one in ten minutes, after the swings and one minute of rest	24kg	48kg

Nikki Shlosser, SFG Team Leader, casually put up 115 reps with a 32kg in five minutes—after dinner with scotch and cake. (PROFESSIONAL DRIVER ON A CLOSED COURSE. DO NOT ATTEMPT.)

The S&S challenge does not offer any breaks for bodyweight or age. This is not an athletic competition, so there is no need for fairness. The way I see it, if you get in a street fight, you will not have the luxury of stepping on a scale or showing your driver's license.

DIE BUT DO

All weakness is a weakness of will.

—Friedrich Nietzsche

Russians have an expression, "Die but do." They amuse themselves comparing it with the American "Do or die." Where a Yankee gets off the hook from fulfilling his orders if he croaks, a Russkie may not use death as an excuse.

There comes a time when training is over and you have got to find out what you are made of. Carl Jung observed, as did many before and after him, "Man needs difficulties; they are necessary for health."

A single set of swings without putting the bell down—what John Brookfield calls "going beyond the interval"—will provide difficulties in spades.

In a normal exercise, a given muscle group or the cardiorespiratory system is the weak link that gives out first. The evil beauty of the swing is, everything is suffering greatly, but nothing gives out first—although you wish it would. One can carry on through sheer willpower.

Brandon Hetzler, a researcher from Missouri State University, describes his five-week trial by swings:

> Another person and I had a swing challenge to 25,000 swings with a 24kg kettlebell. We limited it to 20 minutes per day, five days a week, and made a rig to assure we hit shoulder-level height. Technique-wise, we were both ultra-competitive and were sticklers for perfection. We went for five weeks.

> The first day I did 565 total swings, 265 of them continuous to the 7:15 mark, and it was not pretty.

> Our last day was unlimited time and hand switches, but we couldn't set the bell down. We went 45 minutes straight. I hit 1,800 at that point, and 2,001 at the 49:21 mark. Consciousness came back at 55 minutes—or so I was told.

> I did 165 swings with a pair of 48s in 12 minutes the following week. My grip was ridiculous. My body fat dropped to below 6%, but my weight stayed the same.

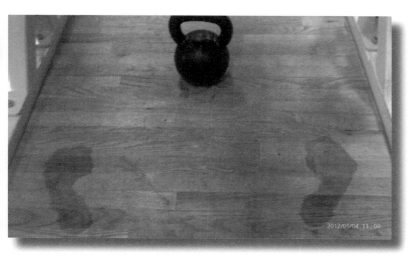

That, ladies and gentlemen, is one harsh way to test your spirit.

Photo courtesy of Brandon Hetzler

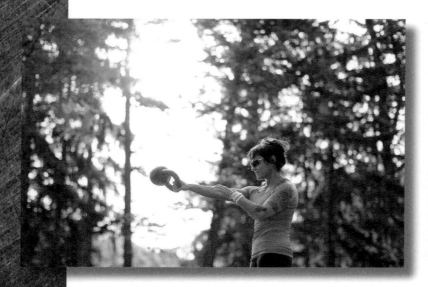
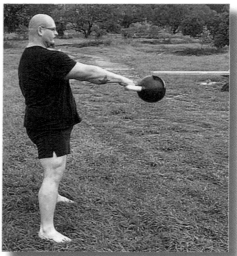

Tracy Reifkind, SFG and Bud Jeffries describe crazy swing quests in their books, **The Swing** *and* **I Will Be Iron**, *respectively.*

Photos courtesy of of Tracy Reifkind and Bud Jeffries

Non-Stop Swing Testing

S&S does not provide you with a program to maximize your non-stop swings numbers. It throws you to the sharks without specific preparation. Naturally, you need your cardiologist's approval.

Every two weeks take a kettlebell one or more sizes lighter than the one you are currently swinging. Pick a swing variation—two-arm, one-arm, hand-to-hand, mixed—and enjoy the pain.

Do not introduce non-stop swings into your training until your normal training weight is 24kg if you are a woman, or 32kg if you are a man. You have no business pushing yourself "beyond the interval" until you have this much strength and experience.

Michael Castrogiovanni, SFG Team Leader, gives a worthy goal to shoot for: 100 non-stop swings, "because it is about the length of a wrestling round." The dual goal is building up the weight to the heaviest possible—48kg for men, 24kg for women—and making it so easy that you can swing it "without breaking a sweat while singing *The Gambler* by Kenny Rogers."

In swing intervals the one-arm swing version is the toughest, whereas in challenges where you do not put the bell down, the two-arm swing might kick your butt harder due to "the rib cage being constricted by fixing both hands to the bell," as Castro pointed out.

I must stress: *The quantity may not come at the expense of quality!*

Review the swing standards; any rep that does not fulfill every one of them is a no-count.

Memorize the speed endurance and hard style laziness chapters.

And watch your breathing like a hawk. Do not reverse your breathing pattern! In other words, do not start inhaling on the way up and exhaling on the way down. Such breathing has its uses, but it is not compatible with maximal power generation.

Take a double sniff of air on the way down—sharply, so your nose gets narrow. It will make a big difference.

The key to safely getting the most out of your trial by swings is treating the set as speed endurance training. Set the goal of maintaining a high speed for as long as possible, as opposed to swinging at all costs.

Catch your bad breath and do your get-ups.

You will be sore the next day. Ignore it and go back to your S&S; it is business as usual.

WRESTLING A KETTLEBELL

- **100 TWO-ARM SWINGS WITHOUT SETTING THE BELL DOWN**
- **EVENTUALLY 24KG FOR LADIES**
- **EVENTUALLY 48KG FOR GENTLEMEN**
- **ANY REP THAT DOES NOT FULFILL EVERY ONE OF THE SWING STANDARDS DOES NOT COUNT.**

In addition, do not be afraid to challenge yourself once or twice a month in a variety of ways. Help a friend move. Shovel snow for the entire block. Take out your dusty boxing gloves and call up your old sparring partners. Run up a mountain with a backpack. Enter a 10K race. Farmer-carry your kettlebells for distance. Take on any physical challenge that will test your spirit without breaking your body.

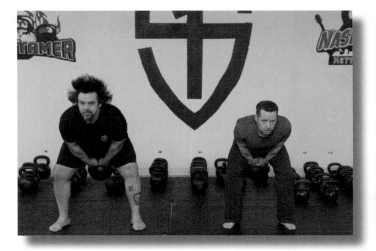
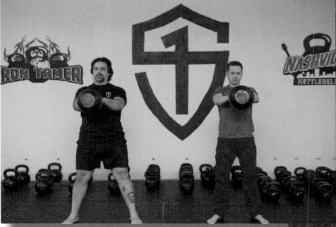

David "Tamer" Whitley, Master SFG calls it "flipping the crazy switch." He and Matt McBryde, SFG Team Leader are taking 48kg "Beasts" for a 1,000 rep ride.

Photo courtesy of David Whitley

Training in a "punch the clock" manner, but always mentally ready to "flip the crazy switch" is for a professional warrior.

A couple of years ago I was talking to my close friend John Faas, a U.S. military special operator who would soon get killed in action in Afghanistan. He was barely thirty, but his body was already beaten up by multiple deployments. He reminded me of the prizefighter in one of O'Henry's short stories: "bony of cheek and jaw, scarred, toughened, broken and reknit, indestructible, grisly, gladiatorial as a hornet…"

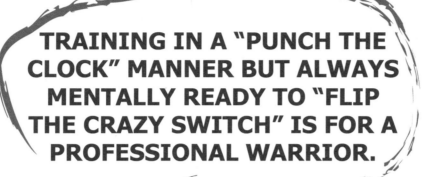

TRAINING IN A "PUNCH THE CLOCK" MANNER BUT ALWAYS MENTALLY READY TO "FLIP THE CRAZY SWITCH" IS FOR A PROFESSIONAL WARRIOR.

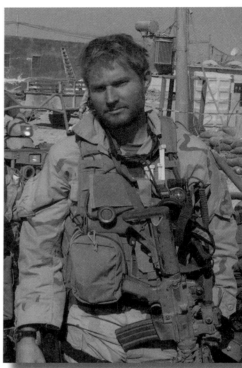

As we were discussing the way he was dealing with his injuries, he summed it up with a line from a country song by Toby Keith: "I'm not as good as I once was, but I am as good once as I ever was."

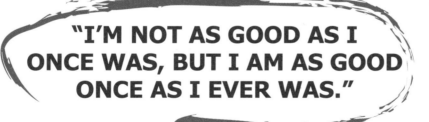

"I'M NOT AS GOOD AS I ONCE WAS, BUT I AM AS GOOD ONCE AS I EVER WAS."

An American hero.
SOC (SEAL Operator, Chief) John Faas.
KIA August 6, 2011, Afghanistan.

Photo courtesy of the Faas family

That was it. The injured sailor was training in a restrained manner, saving himself for when it mattered—in combat. That was the attitude of a professional warrior who had nothing to prove.

A lyrical aside—Marine vet Mark Toomey, Senior SFG, likes to tell eager boys, "Don't try to out-tough professional tough guys." Translation: it does not matter a lick if you can do more swings or run a faster Tough Mudder than a war vet. He has tested his spirit in ways you cannot even imagine, from ruthless selection to facing death over and over. Do not for a second dare to think of yourself as a better man if you have bettered him in some exercise. If the stakes were raised, you know who would come out victorious.

"I am as good once as I ever was."

"DON'T TRY TO OUT-TOUGH PROFESSIONAL TOUGH GUYS."

The swing is a perfect exercise for a Monty Python–type with a strong spirit but a broken body. Bud Jeffries writes:

> The swing allowed me to work around a significant knee injury and a significant shoulder and biceps injury I got from grappling. The swing will allow most people to work around a wide range of injuries or keep going even with "high miles" because it doesn't force you to move into extreme positions. There are a great many exercises that force the body into unnatural positions or to tolerate unnatural amounts of force in unusual ways, or that simply don't work for certain people. The swing, however, creates all the strength benefits and ten times the endurance benefits for most people with little or no pounding on the body. It's very easy on the body and, in fact, is a builder to the body instead of a damager.

Rif is a hard man with high mileage. He is able to test his spirit with swings.

> If you think you are only strong if you can lift a certain number, whatever that number is, you will feel pretty weak most of the time. Strength is not a data point; it's not a number. It's an attitude.

> I've lifted some heavy weights in my life and accomplished some pretty decent feats of strength and endurance. I've also accumulated some serious injuries and put some high miles on this frame. If I only thought of myself as strong relative to what I used to be able to squat, bench or deadlift, or how far I could run, swim, or cycle, I would have to look at myself as being much weaker now than in the past. That would be a mistake, and wrong. I can't lift as much as I used to, but I am stronger than ever.

> No matter how strong you are, there will always be someone stronger than you. Using only a number as the litmus test of whether you are strong or not is self-defeating. You will get older. You will not be able to continue to set personal all-time bests forever. But you can continue to get stronger mentally. You can adjust to whatever the environment is and challenge yourself to push past wherever you are at the moment, in any way you can, and feel good knowing you just made yourself a better man or woman.

"STRENGTH IS NOT A DATA POINT; IT'S NOT A NUMBER. IT'S AN ATTITUDE."

SIMPLE & SINISTER SUMMARIZED

Simplify, simplify.

—Henry David Thoreau

One "simplify" would have sufficed.

—Ralph Waldo Emerson, in response

1. Train daily, taking an occasional day off when your schedule or health prevents you from training. If you follow a serious strength training program, reduce the S&S frequency to twice a week.

2. Start each practice with three circuits of five reps of prying goblet squats, SF hip bridges, and haloes. As an option, follow up with several get-ups with a shoe or a light weight.

3. The main part: 5x10 one-arm swings per arm and 5x1 get-up per arm.

4. Rest actively between sets. Walk around, skip rope, shadow kickbox, shake off the tension, do breathing exercises, do finger extensions with a rubber band.

5. Rest long enough between sets to assure no drop-off in technical proficiency, get-up strength and swing power. Progressively but not aggressively reduce the rest intervals.

6. When you reach the 1:1 work-to-rest ratio in one of the exercises—100 total swings in five minutes; ten total get-ups in ten minutes—and can do this strongly almost any day, move up in weight in that exercise. Gradually replace your current training weight with a heavier weight, one set at a time. Go at your own pace; solidify what you have achieved before going further.

7. Fatigue or stress are no excuse for skipping a training session. Have a light day: reduce the weight in one or both exercises, in all or in some sets. Do two-arm shadow swings with a kettlebell close to 30% of your bodyweight or lighter. In light get-ups, add a ten-second pause at every stage.

8. After the kettlebell practice or later in the day, do one to three sets of passive stretches—the 90/90 stretch and the QL straddle. Hang on a pullup bar if you have one.

9. The "simple" goal for women is 16kg for get-ups and 24kg for swings. The "sinister" goal for ambitious women is 24kg and 32kg, respectively. The "simple" goal for men is 32kg in both events. The "sinister" goal is 48kg. The 10x10 swings must be done in five minutes; the 10x1 get-up in ten minutes after the swings and a one minute rest. A rep that does not fulfill every one of the technique standards is a no-count.

10. Every two weeks take a kettlebell one or more sizes lighter than the one you are currently swinging, and do as many swings as possible without setting the bell down. Pick any swing variation—two-arm, one-arm with multiple hand switches, hand-to-hand, mixed. Any rep that does not fulfill every one of the swing standards is a no-count. After a brief rest, do your usual get-ups. Do not introduce non-stop swings into your training until your normal training weight is 24kg if you are a woman and 32kg if you are a man.

Repeat until strong.

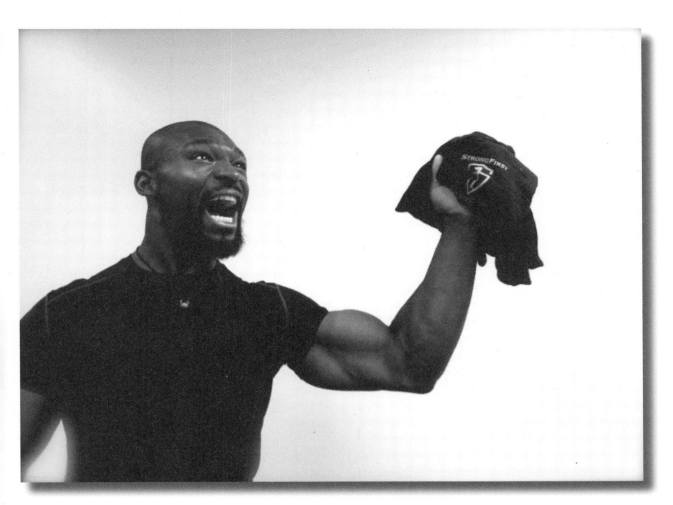

Eugene Kwarteng celebrates earning his SFG instructor diploma.

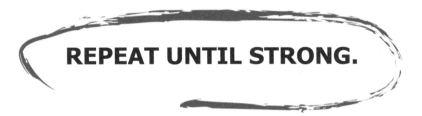

REPEAT UNTIL STRONG.

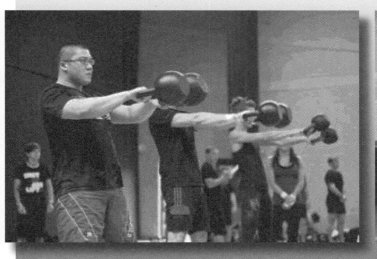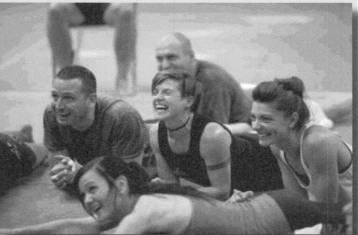

JOIN THE STRONG.

Get the most of your extreme handheld gym—sharpen your kettlebell skills with a StrongFirst certified instructor.

Our worldwide network gives you choices:

- Take **private lessons** or join a **group class**. SFG certified instructors have received the most in-depth education and rigorous testing in the industry and have set the gold standard.

☑ Find a kettlebell instructor

www.strongfirst.com/instructors/

- Take a **one-day course** (no experience required) taught by top StrongFirst certified instructors. Walk away with confidence to train on your own.

☑ Find a one-day kettlebell course

www.strongfirst.com/faqs/sfg-kettlebell-course/

POWER TO YOU!!